POLICE DRUGS

One cannot properly allow oneself to do violence to conscience, and to the inviolable sanctuary of spiritual liberty.—PORTALIS.

POLICE DRUGS

by

JEAN ROLIN

Translated, with a Foreword, by
LAURENCE J. BENDIT
M.A., M.D.(Cantab.), D.P.M.

With an Appendix on Narcoanalysis by
EDWARD V. SAHER

PHILOSOPHICAL LIBRARY
NEW YORK

This is an adaptation of Drogues de Police
published by Librairie Plon, Paris

PUBLISHED 1956, BY PHILOSOPHICAL LIBRARY INC.,
15 EAST 40TH STREET, NEW YORK 16, N.Y.

ALL RIGHTS RESERVED

PRINTED IN GREAT BRITAIN

FOREWORD

THIS book clearly reflects the indignation aroused in many decent French people by one of the scandalous trials which took place after the Liberation, while passions were running high and often affected the course of Justice. But despite its lurid background, it is not out of context with the contemporary scene. On the contrary, it only serves to throw into high relief certain aspects of modern life which exist even under what we have become reconciled to thinking of as normal conditions.

For we live to-day in a world of contradictions, where what the State gives with one hand it takes away with the other. Even in sober, middle-of-the-way Britain, a benevolent Government gives us 'welfare', rehabilitates the disabled and the delinquent, gives each one some positive place in Society, so that his *ego* can have its meed of self-respect. Yet it coerces and dragoons us with forms and enforced insurances, and, moreover, gives each of us at least two code numbers which reduce our private names to secondary place in ministerial files. In some other countries, of course, the individual counts for nothing as against the alleged welfare of the masses, while in others it is the individual who is paramount, and thinks it good citizenship to try and circumvent the laws and regulations made for the sake of Society: but this is only a matter of which way the pendulum has swung in that particular place.

One sign of the times, moreover, is that we are, perhaps more than at any other time, drug-ridden. True, most Governments are concerned in trying to stop the traffic in opium, hashish and cocaine. But their efforts are frustrated by the chemists who, in their laboratories, produce ever new and better—or worse—drugs to stimulate or depress. And in this the medical profession are their accomplices, creating addicts by imprudent prescription—a fact which was recently pointed out in the medical press in connection with those valuable but much abused drugs, the barbiturate group.

True, man has always taken drugs. Whether one craves the humble cup of tea or coffee, or, passing through the field of tobacco and alcohol to that of heroin or morphine, one is in some degree an addict, using the drug to make life pleasanter or even bearable, rather than for some definite medical reason. The ease with which people to-day fall back on their 'sleeping tablets', or on those which have to be taken in the morning to neutralize the doping of the night before (thus taking two poisons instead of one) is one of the more serious problems of the day. But this bad habit is one of people who act freely and not under duress other than that which is self-imposed by allowing the conditions of life to be what they are.

When, however, it comes to a person accused of a crime being in one way or another forced to submit to drugging in order to arrive at the facts of the case, the matter becomes still more serious. It involves the whole question of the relation of man to man, of the collective to the individual. M. Rolin discusses this fully, and it need only be said here that, for the first time, in a recent murder case, evidence of what was said under drug narcosis was allowed in a British Court. The case was one in which the plea was 'Guilty but insane', hence laying on the defence the onus of proving that the prisoner was not morally responsible for the murder with which he was charged. The psychiatrist called in for the defence used what had been said in support of the plea of insanity. This is a very different matter from attempting to extract a confession of guilt, or even to trip the accused into an admission which might compromise him.

The Lancet,[1] under the heading *Nothing but the Truth*, comments on this case, emphasizing that, as a means of finding out actual facts about events, drug narcosis is quite

1. 21 March 1953, p. 585.

unreliable, even to the extent that an innocent person may accuse himself of something which neither he nor anybody else has done. The article goes on to suggest that, pending much more research, as well as consideration of the ethics of the matter, narcosis should only be used (*a*) to diagnose psychosis, (*b*) to diagnose and treat neurosis, (*c*) to distinguish between hysterical and other psychogenic cases and troubles due to genuine epilepsy or organic cerebral injury.

M. Rolin derides the phrase 'truth drug', and with justice as far as facts go. But these drugs do reveal the truth when considered from the psychiatric angle. That is, they bring to light underlying feelings and motives in the patient's mind: things which some primitive part of him *might* like to do, but which, under normal conditions, he would neither do nor perhaps even in his wildest moments think of doing. Yet such is the dramatizing power of the mind when unrestricted and uncensored, that it may result in things being said under narcosis in such a form that it appears as if they were related to things actually done. On the other hand, when fear enters the picture, the story of a crime actually committed is usually kept dark, even under narcosis reinforced by leading questions.

Here the matter stands. But the whole question of drugging shows something of the confusion of the mind of modern man. He seems to have forgotten that the goal of spiritual self-realization is to see 'face to face', and not 'as in a glass darkly', befuddled by drugs, moral or physical. Hence he fills his mind and his body with dope rather than face things as they are. This is an easier thing, no doubt, than to change the conditions he himself has, after all, created, and which he calls fatalistically 'modern life'. So barbiturates, amphetamine, slogans, formulae, ideologies and even religious creeds, are invoked to bolster him up.

What it all amounts to is that man seems to have lost sight of his duty to himself, despite the fact that he is told in the Gospels to 'love his neighbour as himself': i.e., to love himself in the same way as his neighbour. And when that happens, duty to the neighbour becomes obscured. And if one transgresses, the guilt one feels against oneself for not living as one should becomes projected on to him in the form of vindictiveness and cruelty. In this way, all sense of proportion and decency, and hence of equity and justice, vanishes.

All this may seem food for the gloom of those who think the world is going to the dogs. But, from the psychological angle, it is well to realize that the evils of to-day are not new. They have been there all the time. But now—thanks perhaps to Freud and his like—they are no longer suppressed, under the surface, and hence explosive, as they were before our recent pair of world wars. The very fact that hypocrisy and cant are stripped off, and that things appear to-day in their stark ugliness, is a good sign. For it means that they are known and seen, and hence that the first stage towards dealing with them is passed. But it is only when a true sense of morality, based on spiritual intuitions, replaces the false moralities of the past, that peace, justice and happiness will take the place of the present strife, both between men, and, more fundamentally still, within the individual soul.

LAURENCE J. BENDIT.

CONTENTS

CHAP.		PAGE
FOREWORD		v
INTRODUCTION		1
1. THE DEVIL PLAYS APOTHECARY		11
1. Stupefying Drugs		12
2. The Barbiturates		22
3. The Amphetamine Group		29
2. PSYCHIATRIC ASPECTS		35
1. Narco-analysis		35
2. Amphetamine Shock		44
3. THE MEDICO-LEGAL ASPECTS: FROM MEDICINE TO POLICE METHODS		49
1. Diagnosis or Extortion?		49
2. The Process of Deterioration		55
4. THE CENS CASE		69
The Facts		69
5. FORENSIC PRINCIPLES: JUSTICE VERSUS TECHNIQUE		80
1. The Expert's Mandate		80
2. Judicial Examination		87
3. The Paramount Rôle of Legal Principles		90

CONTENTS

CHAP.	PAGE
4. False Science	92
5. The Principle of Inner Conviction	95
6. THE CONFESSION DRUG	101
1. The Nature of the Confession	101
2. Untrue Confessions	107
3. The Prejudice in favour of Confession: The Use of Torture	111
4. A Forensic Criticism of Confession	116
5. The Moral Significance of Confession	119
7. THE SANCTITY OF SECRECY	122
1. The Right to Keep Silent	122
2. The Impenetrable Fortress	128
8. BACKGROUND	135
1. Political	135
2. Justice in Doubt	143
3. Over-confident Medicine	148
4. Justice by Degradation	153
5. Renegade and Martyr	160
6. Truth Serum, Indeed!	164
APPENDIX: NARCOANALYSIS by Edward V. Saher	169

INTRODUCTION

FROM the start, and by using an unambiguous title, I have tried to make entirely clear what I am writing about. Drugs such as pentothal and its companions, which are used in psychological exploration, once they come to be used outside the psychiatric clinic, in connection with courts of law, become simply police drugs. The moment methods of investigating the unconscious pass from the strictly medical and therapeutic sphere into the forensic, these drugs become prostituted into means of extortion, turn the skill of the expert into the work of a policeman, and destroy all chance of true justice being meted out.

I foresee that so categorical a statement will rouse protests among those who want to make a distinction between the use of drugs in making a psychiatric diagnosis for medicolegal purposes and their use in police interrogation. I know and accept that distinction as a hypothesis, and discuss it in such detail that some may think it overweighted, but in the end I have not found it valid. And the strongest reason for my anxiety lies in the attitude which I have met among the experts themselves, in the statements of some, in the acts of others. The advocates of the use of pentothal in the administration of justice have themselves taken care to destroy their own adroit theory of *narco-diagnosis*, and to ensure that there should be no clear demarcation between professional assessment and pure extortion. They actually complain that the warnings given against allowing the police to use such drugs to obtain confessions is the very thing which confuses the mind of the public. In reality the confusion lies only in their own false and vain distinctions.

These distinctions anyway are only made possible by an enormous *a priori* assumption, and by forgetting or passing over in silence a fact which would clarify the whole problem, i.e. the Cens case. Let those who theorize about pentothal and its medico-legal virtues first answer this question: do they know the Cens affair? Do they know how narco-diagnosis was used and what were its results?

In this book, to which I want to give a general significance, I have described the Cens case in the place where a concrete example was required, for it is typical. But it is one which is so overwhelming, that I must own that I was tempted to give it pride of place at the beginning of my book. Was this due to indignation against an abominable miscarriage of justice? Perhaps. But it was also because it showed pentothal in its most lurid rôle. One sees in this case distortion of science hand in glove with prostitution of justice, agreed to persecute a very sick man, hemiplegic, epileptic, aphasic, bed-ridden in a prison cot. One sees an astonishing concourse of physicians, professors, judges, all trying to crush with their considered opinions a poor wretch who dared to ask that some account be taken of three years of preventive detention and misery. Why this great turmoil, with syringes, and legal codes? It was averred that it was for the simple purpose of exposing a malingerer!

For among those who could not hush up the Cens case, either because they themselves were concerned in it, or in order to extricate their friends from it, the argument is still heard that the victim was a malingerer. Even if this were true, I do not see how it justifies the methods used. For how can the exposure of malingering by using a drug which brings about psychic dissociation be called anything but police action? But it is *not* true, Cens was *not* a malingerer. To make this assertion I have no need to give my personal guarantee that he acted in good faith: I do not know him and have never even seen him; I am not his father confessor. I need only refer to medical and legal documents which show that many expert reports, both before and after pentothal narcosis, state that Cens was not simulating incapacity; and the Court of Justice of Toulouse set him free on grounds of ill-health. What weight can one give after this to the rationalizations of experts involved in a nasty business, or to the badly taken points of a judgment where frivolity and iniquity competed?

This is the most famous exploit of pentothal in forensic assessment: the persecution of a genuine invalid as a result of a false diagnosis of malingering. Yet the theorists remain unshaken in telling us of its benefits!

A resounding medico-legal howler: in connection with a *truth serum*. This is indeed strange!

It is high time that this expression, sired by the over-hasty imagination of an American criminologist, should be reconsidered. And I shall think I have done enough in this essay if I contribute to its categorical discredit. But one must be thorough, and this discredit must be final. It is not enough merely to dissipate the illusion of those who think that narcosis provides a genuine technique of interrogation, not enough to point out that pentothal does not abolish the possibility of deceit and lying, that when it makes one 'confess', it usually only produces a muddle of fantasies, delirium, false avowals: in short, that it is only a catharsis of which the truth is just about as great and as valid as that which results from wine drinking. This is not all, however: there is more to say, which is that the Cens case shows conclusively that pentothal is a source of medico-legal mistakes, that it is a drug which leads to false diagnosis and to fallacious answers to questioning. Miscarriage of justice as a result of the duplication of error, that of police methods added to that of medicine: this is what one may expect from this *truth serum*.

Dr. Heuyer sums the matter up very well—and this is no doubt the only point on which we shall be agreed—in the phrase: '*the truth serum is humbug*'. And yet he gave an expert opinion based on this kind of truth.

I expect to be asked what business of mine is all this, I who do not belong to the fold. It is a matter of medical technique, and technicians do not like people to interfere in their affairs. Yet they will have to put up with me.

Let me make myself clear. When I have to speak of a particular technique, I never attempt to mix my own opinions with those of the technicians. I make *them* do the talking and I compare what one says with what others say, and if I make my own judgment, it is based on what I have derived from this. When I say that Dr. Heuyer has made a mistake, I am not merely saying what I believe, I am drawing my conclusions from the opinions of the other experts in the case. When I maintain that narco-analysis will allow medical expert opinion to slide over into police medicine, I do so because of what certain experts are themselves doing or saying. When I affirm that pentothal is an extortive drug, it is as a result of studying the arguments of some of its protagonists in the light of the arguments of others. By thus comparing one side of a question with another, it is within the capacity of every honest man to judge between truth and falsehood. Such judgment is not the prerogative of the technician alone.

Some of these experts refuse to answer for their methods otherwise than at the bar of pure science. This can only be attributed to the claim of autarchy for science, which is one of the most disturbing features of the problem of pentothal. For by this argument it is sought to subordinate the problem to a prejudice in favour of the technical expert. This is one of the poisons of civilization to-day. One of the purposes of this book is to emphasize that technique is not the first consideration, especially as concerns technical methods of mental investigation which are already as formidable, and are soon likely to be as pretentious, as those concerning material things. Without forgetting that only too often one applies the phrase 'technical knowledge' to the hasty conclusions of pseudo-science, the fact remains that technical methods, even when well tried, are not a law unto themselves, but that they must be subordinated to the ends for which they are used.

This principle may easily be forgotten in medicine. In the practice of therapeutic technique the problem scarcely arises, for its purpose, the treatment of the patient, is so evident that it need not be specifically stated. If it is true that the supremacy of this end is safeguarded by the consent of the patient, or those who stand sponsor for him, by the free choice of doctor, and by his right to expect from him a maximum degree of caution and skill, it follows that conflict between the ends to be achieved and the methods used is rare. The close accord, the quasi-identity of ends and means, results in a lack of emphasis on the superiority of the ends to those means.

It is, however, a great mistake to carry this tacit lack of discrimination into the field of forensic medicine, and so conclude that the expert investigator should be given as free a hand in the practice of his art as is allowed the physician at the bedside of his patient, for here the ends are neither so simple nor so obvious. They are, on the contrary, highly complex, and often in dispute: is one here concerned with a straightforward question of diagnosis of health or sickness, or with an assessment of criminal responsibility? with accusing or excusing? with punishment or with therapy? These ends, moreover, are wrapped up in a whole mass of principles of justice and morality on which they are dependent. For the supreme purpose of the law is to render justice, and so belongs to the very bases of civilized life. In view of this and of the complexities it involves, it is clearly most important that the blinkers of technical prejudice should not prevent us from seeing clearly. Medicine is here not the only arbiter of the rectitude of its own methods, for it has to render its account at the bar of justice and hence before the whole community. We are thus in an ambiguous region where different intentions coincide without necessarily agreeing, where men with very different mental habits meet. So it can only be by a philosophical judgment, made from a viewpoint wider than that of any specialist's field, that ends can be determined, and the right subordination of the means to these ends may be decided. Hence, in contradiction to the claims of medico-legal technicians, I set the claims to greater authority on the part of the philosopher and the student of morality.

After this discussion of principles, one has to consider the state of mind of the men among whom these practices take place. I am sorry that certain passages in this book will have to show this in an unpleasant light, but the imperative claims made on behalf of techniques is only too often a disguise for an attempt at dictatorship by the technician. Though the wish to dominate is nothing new, the arrogance of science on the one hand, and the docility of those who submit to it, on the other, allow it to try and justify itself by dubious means. The name of science gives an excellent pretext to scientists who have no doubts—even of themselves—to manipulate, as if by authority, and as if they were simply human guinea-pigs, the people entrusted to their care. We have to-day hospital medicine, administrative medicine, military medicine, statistical medicine: in short, herd medicine. And, while some see the danger of this, are there not many who find a secret satisfaction in it? I do not deny that the insistence of some experts on introducing pentothal into judicial procedure is partly explained by the honourable and genuine wish to add to their powers of diagnosis. But I am afraid that there are others in whom this manifests only a morbid taste for holding at their mercy human material which can only too surely be bent to their will.

I am not at war with doctors as such. But I am opposed to the unbearable pretension to the right to dispose of their fellows which some scientists impudently claim, as soon as their specialized skill invests them with any authority in the social field. This is not mere prejudice. I see it outstandingly in this business of pentothal. I myself, as academician, have stood up against it only recently in the plans for reorganizing certain schools. For it is just the same thing in medicine as in pedagogy when, in the name of technique, one tries to impose on others the dominion of certain ideas—or moods—or fads. Here, certain high priests of the

INTRODUCTION

University make a decree, simply because it suits them, and to the detriment of the essentially spiritual nature of the teacher's function, by introducing reform of the curriculum which proposes to reduce all the children of the country to the level of school-going cattle. There, certain medical pontiffs take the risk of destroying the supremely spiritual significance of their profession and, in the case of pentothal, of upsetting the traditions of justice. This is an attempt to create a general and authoritarian institution, backed if need be by an administrative ukase, to legalize practices which have neither value nor justification otherwise than in a private medical interview. This, of course, applies to the Langevin scheme about the forensic use of drugs.

We have here the evil of a minor tyranny, exercised under the wings of a major one. The ill-founded authoritarianism of corporations such as universities, the medical or legal professions, offer the monster-state the best medium for exercising its domination of the individual. Surrounded from the moment of his birth to that of his death by the triple and insistent vigilance of teacher, doctor and judge, the so-called free citizen has only one course open to him: to conform.

Let us not try and blink the fact: this particular problem covers a field much wider than just that of forensic medicine. Pentothal has come into a world where the soil is well tilled and prepared for the reception of all forms of technique which lead to enslavement and degradation. It is clearly vain to think of its use apart from the social complex of barbarism into which we are sinking.

I quite understand that the experts will be angry at the idea that they can be charged with all that arises out of the base use of drugs by the police; and if I have been deliberately harsh in denouncing the inevitable decadence which is implicit in the logic which justifies their use, I have been very careful not to couple with this any suggestion that those who use them were animated by the evil designs of a torturer. Yet it is a fact that terrifying memories and, worse still, terrifying fears surround the use of pentothal in this manner. They give it an ominous character which its inventors neither sought for nor are prepared to admit. Nevertheless they cannot now rid themselves from the implications.

'Affective states,' said one of these people, with unconscious humour, recognizing the existence of some of these fears, but relegating them to the rank of old wives' tales. I cannot agree, and I have no shame in putting myself in the ranks of those who are indeed moved into an 'affective state' by the present trend of the world. Yes, I am affected by the trial of Cardinal Mindszenty among others. And even if I recognize that there is, fortunately, a large gap between what they did to the Hungarian Primate and what is proposed to us in the form of medico-legal narcoanalysis, I also know that pentothal is only a first step, and that this gap is already bridged by a series of dreadful drugs and horribly exact techniques for bringing about mental breakdown. I can see vistas opening up before us where drugs would have such a prime rôle that I may be excused for feeling certain 'affective states' in anticipation, and at the very thought that even a minor place is already being prepared for them.

Let those who feel themselves immune to such 'affective states' persist in splitting hairs on the distinctions between human rights and forensic medicine, and between narcoanalysis and narco-diagnosis. It is like fiddling while Rome burns or a volcano is about to erupt.

I shall finish this sketch of the basic theme of this essay by pointing out that the use of drugs in psychic investigation raises the matter of one of the most typical aspects of contemporary materialism.

In this century one does not even trouble to label oneself a materialist. One just behaves like one, which is far worse; for if one has to take trouble to deny the existence of Spirit, this is in itself a sign that one is still troubled about whether Spirit exists or not. But when one does not even suspect

INTRODUCTION

that this name may refer to something real, the abuses which materialism leads to are beyond hope of salvation.

Certain advocates of pentothal allege that lumbar punctures and vivisection are admitted and approved, that one uses the reflex hammer and the psycho-galvanometer in neurology. So why pick on this particular intravenous injection for condemnation? The comparison must come as a shock, if one realizes that no real comparison can be made between a purely bodily operation and one which touches on freewill and the integrity of the self. It suggests a form of spiritual rape. But then what can this signify to those who do not even realize that there is such a thing as Spirit, to be capable of being raped?

I confess that it is not easy to determine the exact frontier between ethical operations and those which encroach on the liberty of the individual soul, and violate the secrets of the Spirit. It is not enough to say that this is a matter of feeling, when so many people no longer feel, and since (because it is more effective than the orthodox 'third degree', and causes no *physical* pain, and leaves no traces) there is such connivance over this prostitution of opinion, that confusion is only worse confounded. No doubt it is impossible to find an entirely objective criterion in a field where, when all is said and done, we have to be guided by a form of spiritual tact. I have, however, suggested a rule which appears to shed some light on the problem: one is violating the secrecy of the soul when one tries to break into it directly, and not by observing it indirectly by means of signs and symbols; as soon as one tries to reach the actual source of these symbols and to tamper with the power which governs their expression. An interrogation or an expert assessment can ethically seek only to interpret the signs and symbols which the mind expresses willingly. Any attempt to alter the will of the subject becomes a spiritual assault.

All this really requires more elaboration than I have been able to give in this book—which is, after all, an act of spiritual self-defence and not a thesis for a doctorate in philosophy. The acceptance of the symbol, the respect for a reality behind the symbol—a thing which in itself implies the recognition of this reality—is that not, after all, the basic principle of spiritual philosophy? Going deeper, it is the essential expression of acceptance of the mystery behind religion: *per speculum et in enigmate*. But even without going that far, it must remain the basis of a practical spirituality from which civilized justice cannot depart, if it is careful not to arrogate to itself the right impiously to violate the secret of one's conscience.

I have started this book with a fine passage from Portalis, obviously written in connection with quite another problem—that is, the request made him by Choiseul, to examine the validity of Protestant marriage. But though the subject was different, this passage nevertheless seems magnificently to express the respect which one should preserve for spiritual privacy, and from which one would be loath to see the practice of justice depart.

CHAPTER 1

THE DEVIL PLAYS APOTHECARY

THIS is an old story. It goes back to the times of Noah and his wine. The drunkenness of Noah is the first example of those states of self-abandonment in which, willy-nilly, a man talks of things he would prefer to keep hidden, reveals things which are best not mentioned, gives away his secrets. Because it abolishes self-control and allows unchecked speech, alcohol is clearly the most ancient of those drugs now sometimes spoken of as 'truth serums'.

The Romans coined an ironic proverb which expresses the meaning of this rather tragic collapse of the human mind: *in vino veritas*. It is an irony which tells us much, for it gives a particular value to the word 'truth', used in such a context. It certainly does not mean the truth of the philosopher, which is equivalent to 'the real', and which is consistent all through, but refers rather to a shameless self-exposure, an uncritical giving of confidence, and ill-timed blabbing: a kind of delirium in which a blend of sentimentality, humour, tactlessness, and coarseness give us a picture of people and events—and especially of the principal actor—under a new and surprising light.

Such a consideration seems to have escaped those people who use the phrase 'truth serum', coined in America. If we are to avoid the error of taking it literally, we should never let ourselves lose sight of its relation to the effects of alcohol, for, however diverse may have been the substances which science has produced since the time of Noah, there is still only one way of losing one's wits, and all forms of drugging resemble one another. In short, it would be wrong to expect intoxication, even though produced under the austere wing of science, to be any different from, or less degrading than, that resulting from drinking alcohol; nor should one expect any greater degree of truth to be revealed under the former than under the latter, or that the moral degradation will be any less.

Science, it is true, is working towards what must appear as a more dignified end than mere drunkenness. It invokes to its aid pharmacists, anaesthetists, psychiatrists and criminologists working as a team, and there exists to-day a whole arsenal of drugs, both old and new: a veritable satanic pharmacopoeia. By the use of these, people who are already insane are treated therapeutically, but those who have not yet done so can equally be made to go insane by them.

The same basic principle applies in both cases. In *psychiatry* drugs can help to lift stupor, to break down mutism, and unconscious resistances, and thereby to bring about the objectivization of repressed psychological states, and to allow their analysis. It has been thought that in *criminology* the same drugs would be able forcibly to lift voluntary inhibitions and the controls imposed by consciousness, so as to extract confessions from people who would otherwise refuse to confess, who are lying, or otherwise deceiving their accusers.

Some of these drugs are old and tried natural products, others are the products of man's industry and of recent discoveries in the laboratory. But, disregarding chemical subtleties, we may classify them by their results under three heads: stupefying drugs, barbiturates, and amphetamines.

I. STUPEFYING DRUGS

The action of *hashish*, which is both intoxicating and narcotic, is much like that of alcohol: '*State of waking dream with euphoria, increase of ideation, hypermnesia, logorrhoea*'[1]—'*increase of affect*'. That is, in ordinary words, the subject has more ideas, which come quicker; that he remembers details of events long since forgotten; that he speaks without reticence; that he is more communicative than usual. These facts were made use of as early as 1845, by Moreau, a psychiatrist of Tours, in order to explore the mind and to try and discern unconscious motivations and tendencies.

More recently *Cocaine* has been studied in catatonic states, that is, in conditions of stupor, mutism, and apathy, in an attempt to understand *dementia praecox*.

It does not look as though criminologists have paid proper attention to the results of such research. Only one writer speaks of a strange and already ancient case in which *opium* was used in an attempt to force a confession:

> In 1793, Monteggia, of Milan, despairing of ever sidetracking by ordinary means the dissimulations practised by an admitted criminal, and, because of his being on guard, finding himself unable to make him drunk by means of alcohol, made him take large doses of opium. The victim, barely escaping with his life, *ipso facto* recovered his reason. The indirect success of this heroic form of medication does not, however, seem to have induced the experts to follow Monteggia in this line.[2]

What a strange and brutal wedding of medicine and police procedure! It is a symbol of the ambiguity of such methods: one is left in doubt whether one is trying to unmask a criminal or to heal a sick man. The doubt is not yet resolved, as we shall see later.

Among the more interesting drugs is *mescaline*, an alkaloid obtained from a cactus growing on the high

1. Prof. Divry and Dr. Bobon, of the University of Liège, *La Narco-Analyse au point de vue médico-légal* (*Acta medicinae legalis et socialis*, Brussels, April 1948, p. 602).

2. *Loc. cit.*, pp. 608, 609.

plateaux of Mexico and Texas, *Lophophora Williamsii*,[1] commonly known as *peyotl*.

Among the Mexicans of old, and still to-day among many tribes, 'the devil's root', 'the sacred fungus which intoxicates like wine', is the object of a semi-religious, semi-medical cult, and is used as a panacea. This superstition gave a lot of trouble to the Spanish missionaries of the sixteenth century, who tried to exterminate it. Several handbooks, written for the use of fathers-confessor, advised them to ask some strange-sounding questions, which indicate that peyotl was already used to try and extract secrets and to make the guilty confess. 'Have you eaten peyotl? Have you given any to others in order to find out their secrets, or to discover where stolen objects are hidden?'

The psycho-somatic effects of mescaline have been studied by many people.[2] The strangest of these consist of coloured visual hallucinations, in which the world appears flooded with light and dazzling colour, in disturbance of perception in which movement appears exaggeratedly fast or slow; and in synaesthesia, in which sight and hearing become telescoped: for instance, when the subject hears certain sounds, he also sees certain corresponding colours. These results have been compared with those provoked by hashish, as described by artists, poets, painters, musicians—with particularly susceptible nervous systems.[3] Some

1. Synonyms: *Echinocactus Williamsii, Anhalonium Lewenii*, etc. It is well known that the nomenclature of the cactus family is complex and still indefinite.

2. The literature of peyotl is considerable. The best known work is that of Rouhier, *La Plante qui fait les yeux émerveillés* (Doin, 1935). A more recent one is that of Soulaire, *Cactus et Médecine* (Medical theses, Thiebaut, Paris, 1947). A whole bibliography will be found in them, as well as reproductions of pictures painted under the influence of the drug. [The latest is Aldous Huxley's *The Doors of Perception*, Chatto & Windus, 1954.—*Tr.*]

3. It is known that, in the case of Baudelaire, the poetic doctrine of Correspondences and the psychology of drug effects are closely linked. Even in his normal state Baudelaire speaks of impressions of colour in association with sounds, as, for instance, in *Richard Wagner and Tannhauser*, when he describes his impressions of the prelude to Lohengrin.

writers have even suggested that mescaline intoxication might be used as a psychometric method in bringing into view the latent characteristics of the personality of the subject.

Psychiatrists have tried to study the use of mescaline as a help to mental analysis, especially in cases of dementia praecox.[1]

At the same time as the sympathicomimetic and psychotonic amines were being investigated, mescaline (which belongs to the same chemical family) was used in an attempt to diagnose psychotic cases, but it caused stupefying effects and symptoms of depersonalization, even among normal people, and these obscure psychiatric effects made analysis difficult. It is this very fact, that will-power and the normal control of the personality are inhibited, which criminologists endeavoured to use in order to get confessions. Baroni, in Italy, has thus obtained '*among a few delinquents, at least partial admissions of their acts. Sizaret likewise reports on the case of a sadistic murderer who alternately confessed and denied his crime and who, under the influence of the drug, categorically accused himself of having killed, and described the act in detail.*'[2]

Ten years later, while still in a criminal lunatic asylum, this man still continued to deny the crime.

Mescaline seems to have been used in the camps of Dachau, to weaken the nervous and mental resistance of prisoners during interrogation.

When it comes to *scopolamine* (hyoscine), we are dealing with a drug which has been the subject of much criminological investigation, particularly in the United States, where it has been systematically studied as a means of judicial assessment and of police interrogation. This, indeed, is the 'truth serum', and it is in connection with scopolamine that the term was first launched by Calvin Goddard in 1932, in

1. Mlle. A. Deschamps: *Ether, Cocaïne, Hachisch, Peyotl et Démence Précoce* (Medical theses, Paris, 1932).
2. Divry and Bobon—*loc. cit.*, p. 609.

a series of popular articles on scientific crime detection.[1] Clearly, an expression of only relative accuracy. Scopolamine is not a serum. And, as to truth—we shall discuss this later.

Scopolamine is an alkaloid coming from certain plants of the order of the *solanaceae:* deadly nightshade, henbane, mandrake, of which the stupefying qualities have long been known.[2] From these plants modern pharmacy has extracted atropine, commonly used as an anti-spasmodic (e.g. in coughs and asthma). Scopolamine is a chemical variant of atropine. It is a powerful sedative of the nervous system and is used to control trembling movements, such as that of Parkinson's disease, of St. Vitus' dance, delirium tremens. It is also used as a hypnotic, especially if mixed with chloral, and as an antagonist to morphine in the treatment of drug addiction, because it accelerates the heart-beat and relieves the depression which comes from deprivation. This antagonism is even found valuable when morphine has to be used: the medicine sold under the trade name of *Sedol* is a combination of scopolamine and morphine.

The first one to suggest the value of scopolamine was the American physician, Robert House, of Texas, whose first reports, published in 1897 and 1899, were derived from its use in treating cases of cocaine and morphine addiction. But its psychological effects were first noted when it was used as an analgesic in obstetrics. He tells how in 1916, after delivering a woman under scopolamine analgesia, he conceived the hypothesis which was to turn him towards using it in criminology.[3]

---

1. Calvin Goddard: *How Science Solves Crime*, III. '*Truth Serum*' *or scopolamine in interrogation of criminal suspects* (Hygeia, New York, 1932, p. 337).

2. And is the subject of various fables. It was believed that the root of the mandrake inspired love and made sterile women fertile. Machiavelli wrote a comedy about it, La Fontaine a story.

3. In 1922, in a communication to the Texas Medical Society, and published by the *Texas Medical Journal* (Sept. 1922). My quotation is taken from the reprint of the article in the American Journal of Police Science, after the death of the author in 1930, under the title *Use of Scopolamine in Criminology* (1931, pp. 328 *et seq.*).

THE DEVIL PLAYS APOTHECARY

My attention was first attracted to this peculiar phenomenon, 7 September 1916, while conducting a case of labour under the influence of scopolamine. We desired to weigh the baby, and enquired for the scales. The husband stated that he could not find them. The wife, apparently sound asleep, spoke up and said, 'They are in the kitchen on a nail behind the picture.'[1] The fact that this woman suffered no pain and did not remember when her child was delivered, yet could answer correctly a question she had overheard, appealed to me so strongly that I decided to ascertain if that were in reality another function of scopolamine. In a confinement case, you find your dosage by engaging the patient in conversation, to note the memory test. Hence my investigation was a simple matter. I observed that, without exception, the patient always replied with the truth. The uniqueness of the results obtained from a large number of cases examined was sufficient to prove to me that I could make anyone tell the truth on any question.

On various occasions in his obstetric practice, House noted that, as he talked to his patient with a view to checking the correct dose for analgesia, he got, 'in every case, without exception', true answers to his questions. He thus became certain that he would be able 'to force the truth from any person, on any question'. From this starting point House built up a whole theory as to the influence of scopolamine on the cerebral tissue. He averred that this drug must have the power to interrupt the connection between the centre of ideation on the one hand, and those of hearing and memory on the other. Memory and the power of self-expression remain intact, but superior controls are abolished and the answers given under the influence of the drug must automatically be true. With scopolamine, he says, '*it is impossible to lie*'. This is the origin of the history of scientific methods for extracting confessions.

---

[1]. This refers to a balance with a hook with which one weighs the child wrapped in a blanket. This would explain how it happened that the scales were hanging from a nail.

In subsequent experiments with criminals, House perfected the following technique. He first gave ¼ grain (approximately 15 milligrammes) of morphine with 1/100 grain (approximately 6 milligrammes) of scopolamine subcutaneously. Twenty minutes later, 1/200 grain of scopolamine. Half an hour after, he gave light chloroform anaesthesia. Another thirty minutes later, he gave final injection of 1/400 grain of scopolamine. For the next half hour the subject was ripe for interrogation. House confirmed this by the 'memory test' worked out in his obstetric practice: when he showed the subject a familiar object which he did not recognize and could not name, he was considered to be in the best state for questioning.

House's first experiment took place (let us note the date), on 13 February 1922, in the prison hospital at Dallas, the subject being a man called Scrivener, suspected of two burglaries. Under the influence of the drug he admitted the first but denied the second misdeed. Later on he was proved to be innocent of the latter. This led House to think that scopolamine was a detector of innocence as well as of guilt. This man Scrivener, he told himself, was very intelligent and so enabled the experimenter to document his observations exactly. He notes particularly a very marked hypermnesia, memories apparently lost reappearing very clearly. On the other hand, after the effect of the drug had passed off, amnesia returns and is almost complete, the subject having only a few 'islands of memory' on what has taken place. At House's request, Scrivener wrote his impressions as follows:

> I remember the question, but at the same time I was unconscious of how I answered or of all that I said. After I had regained consciousness I began to realize that at times during the experiment I had a desire to answer any question that I could hear, and it seemed that when a question was asked my mind would enter upon the true facts of the answer and I would speak voluntarily, without any strength of will to manufacture an answer. Well,

doctor, I have not suffered any ill-effects from the experiment, and I feel grateful that I had the opportunity to be of some useful service. Knowing you will be successful in using scopolamine to great advantage, I am ....

Clearly this was a criminal who was interested in the scientific aspects of crime-detection!

While House's experiments in criminology were going on, psychiatrists in the United States were working with narcosis as a means of mental analysis and exploration. In this field, amytal and pentothal gradually took the place of scopolamine. It was psychiatrists who first gave warnings against House's over-confidence in the veracity of statements made under narcosis, and on the impossibility of lying. Evidence of this caution can be found in a communication made as early as 1932 by William F. Lorenz at a meeting of the Chicago Neurological Society, and in the discussion which followed this.[1] Lorenz drew attention to the fact that different people gave different results and suggested that he was far from certain that he was sure when it came to ascertaining guilt. On the other hand, it seems more likely to make sure of innocence. Still more cautious, Dr. Magnus quotes a case of false confession under narcosis, when a patient accused himself of morphinomania and even gave the address of the one who supplied him, both of which statements were subsequently proved untrue. He emphasizes, moreover, that it is easy to obtain confessions of minor misdeeds, but much more difficult to do so if the delinquency is serious—a thing which seems to suggest a remnant of conscious control. Dr. Larson reported that he was present at one of House's experiments when the patient lied consistently all through the sitting!

It was at this point that the judicial question arose. House, who had only been able to carry out his work with the authority of the attorney, wanted the law to approve

---

[1] Lorenz: *Criminal Confessions under Narcosis* (Archives of Neurology, Chicago, 1932, pp. 1221 *et seq.*).

his method of criminal investigation, while at the same time allowing that the patient who refused to submit to it should not be forced to do so. The members of the Chicago Neurological Society were more cautious. Lorenz considers that it is not the physician's place to conduct the enquiry. He should only make sure that the health of the person is such as to make the injection safe, and, if so, to put the patient into the proper state of narcosis and then to withdraw, leaving the matter of the interrogation to the prosecuting attorney or the special investigator. One's mind turns to the physician of olden days who looked after the medical aspects of the torture chamber. Dr. Meyer Solomon is more definite: the use of narcosis in criminal cases, especially without consent, or with the victim unprepared, is a proceeding directly contrary to the true nature of the relationship between the physician and his patient.

Is 'confession under narcosis' current practice in the United States? It is difficult to know. American policemen have a decided liking for allegedly scientific methods which aim directly at the mind of the patient, as a means of forcing a confession. (Typical of these is the 'lie detector', also called the polygraph. This is a collection of recording apparatus designed to show physiological disturbances from emotional causes, and in particular those which are caused by lying. A pneumograph notes any change of respiratory rhythm, a cardiograph that of the pulse. Another part measures the psycho-galvanic reflex—i.e. the change in the electrical resistance of the skin when sweat is secreted.) In this, they are very different from our own scientific policemen, who are more inclined to study traces and marks such as finger-prints, blood, hair, etc., from a physico-chemical angle. Has the 'truth serum' really been added to the scientific equipment of American police?

I have before me a popular magazine wherein an article,[1] with case reports and photographs, seems to indicate it

1. David Dressler: *The Drug That Makes Criminals Talk* (*Saturday Evening Post*, 27 Dec. 1947).

is commonly used, and that public opinion is now accustomed to the idea. But the text of the article itself is better than its lurid title and the disgraceful illustrations at first led one to suppose. It speaks with proper reserve about the efficiency of the drug, which is often found to mislead. It also casts doubts on the legality of the procedure, pointing out that it would be a breach of the Constitution of the United States to use it without the patient's consent—a fact which accounts for the few cases in which it is actually applied. In general, this article emphasizes that pentothal should properly be used mainly in psychiatry, for the treatment of amnesia and neurosis.

I must add, moreover, that one of my friends, having put a direct question to the Federal Bureau of Investigation, and asked to be documented on the use of narcosis in judicial enquiries, received the following answer, signed by its chief:

> Your letter of 25 February 1949, has been received. Although I would like to be of service, this Bureau does not have any information available for distribution of the type you requested. For your information, techniques of this nature are not used in the investigations conducted by the FBI. It is suggested that you may wish to contact the reference librarian of the New York Public Library for information such as you desire.

The head of the Abbott Research Laboratories, the firm who make pentothal, gave a still more interesting answer. He began by giving a large amount of psychiatric references on the use of pentothal. After a second enquiry from my friend, he wrote:

> In answer to your recent letter we regret exceedingly that we do not understand what is desired by your request for literature and experiences 'in the utilization of pentothal in judiciary practice'.

Is this discretion an indication of virtue? I think rather that the 'truth serum' has in the past had a lot of attention in America, and that we are beginning to be interested in it only as they, on the contrary, are giving it up.

2. THE BARBITURATES

Let us come back to pentothal, on which we have anticipated, in order to complete our American story. If scopolamine is an alkaloid, that is, a vegetable product, pentothal is a substance produced in the laboratory. And if it is true that the use of scopolamine in anaesthesia first suggested its psychological effects, this was coincidental. Pentothal, on the other hand, was born of a whole mass of research into the production and nature of artificial sleep.

The principles are well known: during anaesthesia the subject goes through two intermediate phases, one before and one after the deep stage. During these, having lost the upper levels of control, but being quite able to speak, he may bring out some of the contents of the unconscious mind from a greater or a lesser depth which, in full conscious control, would remain suppressed. Under these conditions people blurt out their secrets, own up to hidden actions, give vent to feelings which until then they have controlled and concealed. We know, for instance, of a husband who confessed to infidelity in a way which did not improve his home life, and another where the patient, despite his conscious efforts at reticence, was unable to prevent himself from uttering words which he knew would cause pain to one of his close intimates who was there as he came round. It is even said that certain surgeons had the embarrassing experience of hearing against their will of a crime committed by their patient.

This relaxation of voluntary control and the bringing to the surface of deeper mental levels did not fail to attract the attention of psychiatrists, and suggested to them the use of the twilight stage, whether before or after deep anaesthesia, with a view to exploring morbid psychological states.

Ether was, of course, the first drug used, and one has to go back to 1854 to find the first researches by Morel into the post-narcotic phase of ether anaesthesia.

Affective states which had been forgotten return to

consciousness; traumatic sexual events and tendencies come to light; mutism and the stupor of melancholia may break down, and so give access to a psychic level otherwise unapproachable.

This method is still used to-day by psychiatrists as an aid to analysis, because ether brings about moments of lucidity and recovery of memory.

In criminal cases, Morel used ether without obtaining any confessions. In 1938, a German psychiatrist who used it got 'such fantastic confessions that he refused to credit them in any way'.[1]

Hypnosis, which, as we know, has been the subject of very much research by Charcot and Bernheim, and has been very much talked about, can be compared with ether narcosis. If this method of inducing sleep has been largely replaced by chemical anaesthetics, it is because it was shown to be full of risk such as over-suggestibility, as well as having only a limited scope because the psychic resistances of the subject remained intact. It is generally recognized that it is impossible to make a hypnotized person perform any action contrary to his deeper tendencies and even to his usual normal habits. Nor is it possible to analyse anybody who resists such analysis.[2] This is why hypnotism has had only an ephemeral and slightly ridiculous history in the annals of criminology. It boils down to a suggestion by a German psychiatrist that an accused person and even witnesses in a case should be hypnotized, and a case in Tulle concerning anonymous letters, in which an examining magistrate[3] who used hypnosis in his chambers, produced no other effect than that of bringing about his own dismissal.

1. Divry and Bobon, *loc. cit.*, pp. 603 and 609.
2. Divry and Bobon, *loc. cit.*, p. 608.
3. *Juge d'instruction:* there is no such official in British Courts. He is a judicial officer working in chambers to draw up a *prima facie* case. In Britain the equivalent rôle is played in the first instance by the police, and in the second by the magistrate in open Court when considering the committal of a prisoner to a higher Court. —*Tr.*

POLICE DRUGS

It is by the use of *barbiturates* that it was hoped to work out an accurate technique of psychiatric narcosis.

This class of drug is well enough known because of the many varieties provided by commercial manufacturers: gardenal, veronal, dial, etc. There is consequently no need to give the reader a lesson in chemistry. At the same time, it must be pointed out that all of them are derivatives of barbituric acid, otherwise called *malonyl-urea* (the result of the action of malonic acid on urea), and that the number of these derivatives is legion, according to the different values which these two radicals have in any combination. The constitution of the radicals is, moreover, very important, in that it is that which determines the hypnotic action of the particular variety. It is relatively simple for drugs in common use, such as veronal and gardenal,[1] but it becomes progressively more complex in those chief drugs used for anaesthesia, i.e. *amytal*, *evipan* and *pentothal*. This last has the special property of having a sulphur atom in the place of oxygen in the urea radicle, which makes it a derivation of *thio*-urea: a thio-barbiturate.[2]

---

1. The English name for this is the well-known and much overprescribed Phenobarbitone.—L.J.B.

2. Scientific jargon would be out of place in this book. A general chemical formula will, however, enable us to grasp the principle more easily. The formula of the barbiturates is as follows:

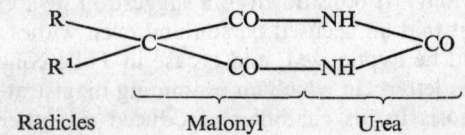

$$R\diagdown_{\diagdown}\diagup^{CO-NH}\diagdown$$
$$CCO$$
$$R^1\diagup^{\diagup}\diagdown_{CO-NH}\diagup$$

   Radicles   Malonyl   Urea

In the drug series, the radicles $R+R^1$ become increasingly complex. Thus we have:

   Veronal: *di-ethyl*—malonyl-urea.
   Gardenal: *phenyl-ethyl*—malonyl-urea.
   Amytal: *iso-amyl-ethyl*—malonyl-urea.
   Evipan (or Hexobarbitone):
          methyl-1-2-*cyclo-hexenyl-methyl*—malonyl-urea.
   Pentothal: *ethyl*-5 (1 *methyl-butyl*)—thio-malonyl-urea (thio= CS instead of CO in the urea formula above).

Barbiturates as a class are weak acids and only slightly soluble in water. Their very soluble sodium salts are those mostly used in practice. The precise names of those are *sodium amytal*, *evipan* (officially *Hexobarbitonum Solubile B.P.*). The Trade names for these are various and depend on the manufacturer. Thus sodium evipan is called *privenal* by one firm, *narconumal* by another. Pentothal sodium is sold in America as *pentothal Abbott*, in France as *nesdonal* and as *anaesthetic* 245 *R.P.*

Pentothal sodium is a white powder, unstable in the presence of oxygen, and so is sold in a sealed ampoule accompanied by another ampoule of double-distilled water in which to dissolve it. The solution must be freshly made and used at once, or it deteriorates within half an hour. It is given by intravenous injection, a certain quantity at a time, each dose being carefully measured and timed, according to the depth and duration of anaesthesia which is desired. It follows that the exact technique varies according to whether one is using it for long or short surgical operations, or for psychiatric narcosis. We shall give further details of the latter later on.

The effects of small doses of the barbiturates are familiar. They are sedatives and hypnotics, quieting anxiety, restoring sleep in cases of excitement or depression. In larger doses they produce anaesthesia. In still higher doses the vital centres are affected and coma and death ensue. They are often used by suicides.

It was in surgery that the method of using pentothal and its analogues was perfected, in 1931 in Germany, in 1933 in France.[1] It is important for us to notice that these drugs, which are so dangerous because of their possible misuse, are valuable friends where surgery is concerned, for they are anaesthetics with a great range of application owing to the wide margin between the normal and the lethal dose. The latter is as much as three to four times greater than the

1. It was used in other countries, including Britain, at about the same time.—*Tr.*

former. They are almost non-toxic for, if the liver is functioning normally, they are rapidly destroyed in the body, and there are no effects from accumulation of them in the system. They avoid the unpleasantness to the patient of the anaesthetic mask, and of the first breaths of ether or chloroform, and they suppress all pre-operational anxiety, replacing it by calm and a feeling of well-being. After the operation, too, they produce forgetfulness and, besides, avoid the serious discomforts which follow the use of volatile anaesthetics. They can be used in all operations, either as a starter, after which anaesthesia is carried on with some other drug, or as a basal local anaesthetic,[1] and are equally good for short operations as for long ones lasting for as much as five or six hours. They are contra-indicated only in cases where liver function is markedly deficient, and in operations in the region of the larynx and the pharynx, where they abolish the reflexes. Finally, it is reported that the effects of the anaesthetics are variable and very individual. There is no absolute standard of dosage.

What makes it fashionable [writes Dr. Forgue, about sodium evipan] are its qualities of euphoric narcosis and the absence of all psychic shock, that it is harmless to the principal organs, particularly to the respiratory system, and that it is quickly disintegrated and eliminated. It is also because of its multiple uses when given by the intravenous route: it is a polyvalent drug, a general servant, good for basal narcosis, for temporary anaesthesia in minor surgery and, because of the possibility of spacing out the doses so as to avoid all risk of giving an overdose, for complete and prolonged anaesthesia in major operations.[2]

---

[1]. That is, to produce unconsciousness, but not the deep muscular relaxation often required. The latter is nowadays brought about by the use of Curare or some other substance.—*Tr.*

[2]. Forgue: *Précis d'anesthesie chirurgicale* (Doin, 1942). I must add, in truth, that not all the anaesthetists I have asked are as positive as this. Some are afraid of asphyxia from laryngeal spasm. I note particularly a communication from Drs. Rudolf and Loo on a case of

Pentothal and its brothers are thus two-faced friends, like all the other discoveries of modern science. The best of them can be used for the worst purposes. I have spoken of the benefits first.

With the exception of the method of treatment known as 'prolonged narcosis', used since last century by psychiatrists in certain cases, the use of barbiturates in mental disease goes back only to 1930. At this date an American psychiatrist, Bleckwenn, brought about, in a case of dementia praecox, a moment of lucidity during narcosis, which made mental exploration possible. One of his co-workers, in 1936, quoted before the Chicago Neurological Society, 'the case of a catatonic who, for two years, was able to feed himself adequately and to write his autobiography, thanks to the lucid intervals brought about by the daily injection of sodium amytal'.[1] In England, the chief promoter was Horsley, who used pentothal as a means of analysis. That is, he made use of its properties of inhibiting cortical control to allow the revelation in consciousness of hidden ideas and feelings. In 1936 he launched the term *narco-analysis*, thereby linking this method with that of Freudian psychoanalysis. He gathered together the results of his work in the form of a book[2] which is the first complete monograph to be published on this subject.

The same method was to gain ground through American army psychiatrists in North Africa, who used it from 1942 onward in the treatment of war neurosis ensuing from emotional shock, especially among airmen. Narcosis was used at that time for the dual purpose of analysis, to bring back repressed emotions and memories to the patient's

polyneuritis after anaesthesia from 3.80 grammes of privenal in which, after coma lasting three days, then five days without symptoms, polyneuritis set in which was not entirely cured after eight months in hospital. The writers are agreed that it is wise 'to be careful of the doses used with the aim of producing long periods of anaesthesia' (*Annales Médico-psychologiques*, 12 Jan. 1946, p. 177).

1. Divry and Bobon, *op. cit.*, p. 605.
2. Horsley: *Narco-Analysis* (Oxford University Press, 1943).

consciousness, and also in order to diminish manifestations of fear.

Although evipan sodium was used in France as early as 1934 by Dr. Justin-Besançon, it was the work of the American army psychiatrists which really introduced the practice of narcosis into France. Since 1943, these names occur: Dr. Sutter, in the Algerian forces, Professor Delay and his colleagues at Sainte-Anne, Dr. Heuyer at Necker (sick children), Dr. Cossa and his co-workers in Nice, Professors Cornil and Ollivier in Marseilles. The method is to-day commonly practised by all psychiatrists, with varying degrees of confidence and of frequency.

As we have seen, the use of barbiturate narcosis in criminology was first mooted in America in 1932, following the use of scopolamine; and Lorenz's communication to the Chicago Neurological Society already voiced a number of reservations on both the authenticity and the legality of any confessions obtained by them. The question is still unsolved. For even though they may agree on the fact that the phrase 'truth serum' is a serious exaggeration, medico-legal specialists are divided on the question of the confessions themselves. Some speak of the valid confessions they have obtained, and others say one gets nothing of the sort, but that narcosis is only ethical as a help in making a diagnosis of the mental state of the subject. It is in this guise that the matter was laid before the French Medico-legal Society in 1946, only to be brought into prominence in 1948 in a judicial *cause célèbre*. This is, indeed, the key subject of this book.

Is it indeed possible to calculate exactly what are the psychological effects of barbiturates, and to diagnose the mental condition of the patient under narcosis? Opinions are mixed, and this diversity is doubtless due to the variable influence of each drug on different individuals. We shall have occasion to return to this question several times in the course of what follows. But this much can be stated at once, that, despite seemingly contradictory observations, there is generally agreement that conscious control is always more or less abrogated, that self-consciousness and the power of self-criticism are sometimes diminished, but sometimes remain intact. Suggestibility and lucidity in interrogation are in some cases very marked, at other times the psychological defences remain unshaken. Sometimes the subject confesses, at other times he does not. The most certain thing is that a state of mental disequilibrium occurs, and that in it shyness and suspiciousness are lessened, 'affective contact'—i.e., mental sympathy and the wish to confide—is increased, together with the desire to externalize thoughts and feelings. In short, the over-all effect is one of 'euphoric catharsis'.

3. THE AMPHETAMINE GROUP

This is a group of drugs of an entirely different chemical nature from the former. Their results are still more astonishing and disturbing.

Everybody knows the name of *ephedrine*, the alkaloid obtained from *Ephedra Vulgaris*. It is used in every patent remedy for its property of relieving congestion and so palliating if not curing the inflamed mucous membrane of the nose in the common cold. Ephedrine is the prototype of the Amines which act on the sympathetic nervous system, whether it be administered by mouth or by injection, it produces a powerful vaso-constrictor and broncho-dilator effect, it brings about a marked and lasting rise in blood-pressure, and it stimulates respiration.

Among this group of amines are some which have also a stimulating effect on the central nervous system and act psychotonically. To some extent ephedrine itself does this, and already in 1913 it was recognized that it caused insomnia, so that some physicians used it in the treatment of narcolepsy, or pathological sleep. But it was a derivative of ephedrine, phenyl-iso-propylamine sulphate (also called phenyl-i-amino-2-propane, or *amphetamine*), which first brought into prominence its dual action on both the sympathetic and the cerebral systems.

Amphetamine is known in the trade by various names: *Benzedrine, Phenedrine, Ortedrine*. It is a substance in the molecule of which there is an asymmetric carbon atom—i.e. one in which each of the four valencies is connected with a different radicle. The result is that one may have two optical isomers of the same chemical molecule with different properties. These can be distinguished in the laboratory by the fact that one of them rotates the plane of polarized light to the right, the other to the left. A mixture of these dextro-rotatory and laevo-rotatory molecules, usually to be found in equal quantities, is called *racemic* and does not affect polarized light.

The first work on the rotation of polarized light was done by Pasteur, beginning with tartaric acid, and later with the sugars.

> They were the basis of all his work. Some living creatures can, under certain conditions, distinguish between the isomers in a particular substance. Some bacteria will cause fermentation of only one of the isomers in a given sugar. Practically all the amino-acids of animal and vegetable protein are dextro-rotatory isomers. In pharmacy, adrenaline is a familiar example. Pasteur emphasized these facts, as far as they were known in his day, and saw in them one of the essential characters of life—i.e. the need for a certain asymmetry of chemical structure. The pharmacology of the derivatives of ephedrine confirm this. The common preparations of them (e.g. amphetamine) are actually racemic mixtures. If one isolates the optical isomers, one realizes that action on the sympathetic belongs to the laevo-rotatory isomers, that on the brain to the dextro-rotatory.[1]

This dextro-rotatory form of amphetamine, used most commonly in the form of *methyl-amphetamine chloride* is

---

1. L. G.: *La méthyl-amphétamine dextrogyre en psychiatrie* (Journal des praticiens, 1 July 1948, p. 322).

sold by different manufacturers of drugs, under different names. In 1938, the Germans called it *Pervitine*. In 1940, a British firm launched it as *Metedrine*. In the United States it is *Desoxine*, in France the well-known *Maxiton* (actually a tartrate; another special preparation, *Kinortine* is also a tartrate, *mixed with caffeine*).

The various salts (chloride, sulphate, etc.) of methylamphetamine are white powders, stable in air, slightly soluble in water, non-hygroscopic. They can be given by mouth (in tablets of 3 to 5 milligrammes), subcutaneously, intramuscularly, or intravenously, according to the intensity and the rapidity of the action sought for.[1]

The average dose is 10 mgm., though higher doses may reach 15 mgm. '*We have*,' says Professor Delay, '*suggested the term* amphetamine shock *to describe the intense and violent results of intravenous injection of* 15 *mgm. of methyl amphetamine.*'[2]

The same author gives a picture of the psychophysiological results which follow the administration of a medium dose of 10 mgm. by mouth. At the affective level it brings about euphoria, increased activity, a greater urge both to work and to talk. At the intellectual level, the result is an increase in intensity and consecutiveness of ideation, and a resistance to sleep. It is not clear whether the added intellectual efficiency is not secondary to a happier affective attitude towards the task in front of one, so that it is not established that the drug has any direct influence on the intelligence. At the physical level, fatigue vanishes, performance increases, muscular effort becomes more powerful and more sustained. In the last war, the German army used

[1]. Delay, etc.: *Étude comparée de l'action psycho-physiologique des divers amphétaminiques dextrogyre et racémique* (Semaine des hôpitaux, 14 Sept. 1948).

[2]. Delay, etc.: *Le choc amphétaminique*. (Communication made to the Medical Society of the Hospitals of Paris, 12 March 1948. Published in the Bulletin of the Society, Nos. 9, 10, 11, p. 308. Masson, publishers.)

pervitine extensively with its shock troops, armoured units, parachutists, and with airmen principally to offset the loss of efficiency at high altitudes. Among normal people the middle range of doses, of from 5 to 10 mgm., does not appreciably affect either breathing, temperature or pulse. The effect lasts about ten hours.

The shock dose (15 mgm.) produces much more violent reactions.

From the psychological angle we have provoked in several normal people a state next door to hypomania, with extreme volubility, a sense of power and euphoria. Arterial pressure rises from 40 to 50 millimetres in 10 to 15 minutes. Breathing becomes deep, motor activity is often marked. In one case a normal person produced an acute display of anxiety.[1]

The indications for using methyl-amphetamine are many. In case of emergency, where intense physical or mental work is required, it combats fatigue and the desire to sleep. It is used in physical and psychic depressive conditions, in post-operative shock, in the depression which comes after infectious illnesses. It subdues the pangs of hunger (and, in large doses, produces anorexia and inanition), despite the increase of bodily activity, and so is used in the treatment of obesity. It helps the treatment of drug addiction, such as that for morphine or tobacco, by avoiding the painful sensations and depression resulting from sudden deprivation. Methyl amphetamine is also used in the treatment of drunkenness. It brings about a spectacular recovery from alcoholic coma. In paediatrics it is used to combat lack of concentration and to calm down restlessness. In psychiatry, the use of amphetamine for exploring and treating psychoses and neuroses is still going on and will be referred to later.

The most outstanding results are to be found in the treatment of narcolepsy.[2] It is much more effective than

1. Delay, etc. : *op. cit.*, p. 315.
2. Justin-Besançon: *Le traitement du coma barbiturique par le phényl-1-amino-2-propane* (Soc. Médicale des Hôpitaux de Paris, 12 Mar. 1948, Bulletin No. 9.10.4, p. 305).

ephedrine or strychnine in coma from an overdose of barbiturates, and the margin of safety allows large doses to be used. With it one often gets an immediate return to consciousness, and if the treatment has been given prior to the occurrence of irreversible nervous lesions or pulmonary complications, the cure can become complete. The antagonistic actions of barbiturates and the amphetamines is used regularly in psychiatric practice, and we shall see that this is perhaps the most worrying aspect of the matter, because of the strange psychological results of the conjoint use of the two drugs.

Is methyl amphetamine a poison? The lethal dose for man is not known, though a massive amount of 200 mgm. produced violent agitation, fainting, nausea, vomiting and palpitation.

The question arises whether there is danger of addiction among those who receive small doses over a long period. Strictly speaking there is not: neither is there accumulation in the tissues, nor does it lose its physiological powers, nor are there any serious difficulties, as there are with morphine, as a result of deprivation. Nevertheless, there are people who make a habit of using methyl-amphetamine, '*to increase their activity, and who have progressively to increase the dose to compensate for the fatigue due to their increased activity and to insomnia*'.[1] They thus enter a dangerous vicious circle: fatigue grows, doses have to be increased, and soon, it seems likely, it is the cause of the state of agitation with depression so well known to students who have overindulged in the drug before their examinations.

In conclusion, let us emphasize that the absorption of large quantities of these drugs over a long period can produce a real toxic psychosis: a hallucinatory delirium of a paranoid type, coupled with anxiety.

To sum up: the psychological effects of the amphetamine group are most characteristically a state of mind divided or polarized between two opposite terms, i.e., euphoria and

1. Delay, etc.: *op. cit.*, p. 319.

anxiety. Yet there is no clear line of demarcation between these. The euphoria from small doses is typical: no less so than the anxiety from large doses. Yet it appears that both the euphoria and the fear interpenetrate one another in a curious manner. Here is how a friend describes his feelings, as a result of taking *Maxiton* in normal doses, for the purpose of intensifying his intellectual work:

> Abnormal lucidity in the organization and promotion of ideas. Everything arranges and classifies itself, things link up and deductions follow with the speed and momentum of a *logical delirium*. In the background there is a shadow of anxiety: the spirit feels itself being carried away willy-nilly and wonders where it will stop.

Anxious euphoria, euphoric anxiety: I will allow myself the risk of using these paradoxical terms to describe the typical effects of methyl-amphetamine, the last arrival into the pharmacists' inferno.

CHAPTER 2

PSYCHIATRIC ASPECTS

THE legalistic problem as regards drugs arises from the fact that their use in forensic medicine as a means of diagnosis of mental conditions among suspected criminals, was first suggested by their use in psychiatry, both for the diagnosis and the treatment of the sick. It is therefore right that I should make clear the medical side of the matter.

1. NARCO-ANALYSIS

This name is given to psychological analysis carried out by a psychiatrist on a patient in whom conscious control and unconscious censorship are inhibited by semi-anaesthesia. Here are some of the technical points concerning it.

Three barbiturates are most frequently used by psychiatrists, and each has its own properties. *Pentothal* is quickly diffused throughout the body, and quickly gives a hypnogogic state of considerable depth, but not of long duration. It needs to be handled very slowly and cautiously, because it has occasionally, though rarely, produced fatal syncope by its action on the vagal system. *Evipan*, still more easily diffused, produces sudden anaesthesia, but often with manifestations of excitement which hinder analysis. *Amytal* is less quickly diffused but rapidly disintegrates in the system. It is, however, free from the defects of the others, and so is preferred by some specialists.[1]

The suitable dose varies widely, according to the patient. As a general rule the drug is given intravenously in a 2.5%

1. Cornil and Ollivier, *Etudes de neuro-psycho-pathologie infantile* (2nd booklet. Committee for the care of Abnormal Children, Marseilles, 1948). Reference can also be made to many other books and articles.

solution (8% for amytal) at the rate of 1 c.c. per minute, up to a total of 6 c.c. (8 c.c. for amytal). In this way the narcosis comes on gradually and reaches a hypnogogic level just before complete unconsciousness. If the dose is larger, or more rapidly injected, the patient goes into full anaesthesia lasting ten minutes or so. One can thus dispose of a choice of two phases for one's attempted exploration: one in the twilight state before anaesthesia, one in that before full consciousness returns. In either of these, the psychological reaction of the patient may vary a lot. Sometimes he may day-dream spontaneously, more often he has to be questioned. He may also refuse to speak and remain on the defensive, while he may equally become very suggestible and amenable. With amytal the hypnogogic state is deep and much effort is needed to keep the patient awake by means of questions. With pentothal sleep is not so near, but the patient's psychic resistance is greater despite a greater loquacity. If one wants to accentuate the hypnogogic state without allowing sleep, one uses strychnine or vitamin B6, or methyl-amphetamine as an antidote. This more complex procedure gives some measure of control of the degree of relaxation, so that one can find the best conditions for the analytical purpose at which one is aiming.

Precautions are, however, necessary. The prior injection of atropine in vago-tonic cases is an instance, if one wants to avoid syncope. It is necessary too to watch the rhythm of the breath and the pulse, and to avoid any sudden fall of blood-pressure. After the session, too, one has to be sure that the patient goes to sleep naturally, and not as a result of an accumulation of barbiturates. Strychnine must be on hand in case a sudden crisis demands quick awakening, as must a carbon dioxide cylinder in case artificial respiration is called for. In short, the whole outfit for resuscitation in case of collapse, is required.[1]

1. Cornil and Ollivier, *op. cit.*, p. 13. These precautions are advocated especially where narco-analysis is used on children. But it seems useful to note them as a matter of general importance.

PSYCHIATRIC ASPECTS

Contra-indications to the method are where there is high blood-pressure, during convalescence from acute illness, when the liver is deficient and when there is idiosyncrasy towards the barbiturates.

Obviously, narco-analysis should not be undertaken too light-heartedly. It should be realized that, though the actual technique of narco-analysis is a recent and special development, the background to it is not new. It is simply one part of modern psychiatric research, all of which is directed towards the destruction of unhealthy mental attitudes and their replacement by healthy ones. Narco-analysis is, in effect, an extension of Freudian psycho-analytical technique.

Mental exploration under narcosis differs fundamentally from psycho-analysis in that it obtains by the use of drugs a form of co-operation from the patient which the Freudian method obtains only by the use of his own free-will. Nevertheless the principle remains the same, to circumvent, in the one case by consent, in the other by a form of constraint due to the power of the drug, the factors which prevent the rise of repressed mental contents into consciousness. These contents, repressed or blacked-out by fear, are the cause of mental troubles, of which the actual illness is a symbol or an indirect expression; and if the unconscious complexes of conflicting thoughts and feelings are allowed to come into the light of day, cure should result.

It is obvious—and it is for the reader to decide whether this is a strength or a weakness—that most practitioners link narco-analysis to the Freudian doctrine of mental life, and their language is that of psycho-analysis.

One aims at reaching a 'half-way state' in which the subject is set free from social rules and conventions imposed by community life and education. These conventional attitudes grow out of conscious or unconscious internal conflict and are the root of repressed tendencies and of the conditions which complicate them. In this half-way state the will weakens, the vigilance of the fully conscious mind diminishes, 'censorship' vanishes. The patient shows himself as he is—or rather, as he ought to be if he were unrestrained. He has an irresistible desire to talk, to confide, to publicize his introspections. He no longer hides behind the mask of the personality which he wears on the stage of Society. Shyness, reticence, shame, are overcome. The real face of the person is exposed. He drops all disguises, his unconscious stands bare and he shows the doctor his real self. It is in this more or less free period that repressions of which the patient is usually quite unconscious come to the surface.

This is the time 'ripe for confession, for spontaneous admissions, for affective transference'.[1] It is then that a *rapprochement* takes place between patient and doctor. . . . During the ensuing talk, sometimes spontaneously, sometimes as a result of laborious evocation . . . many psychic mechanisms . . . repressed by the conscious mind, show themselves. These have been relegated to the unconscious field because they were not in accord with the accepted tenets of social life. The part played by these repressions in the genesis of neurosis is well known, and the symptoms vanish as soon as the unconscious happenings stop being unconscious.[2]

After the analytical phase, synthesis follows:[3]

to help the patient to integrate in consciousness the memories exhumed from the unconscious—to guide him in the reconstruction of a personality set free from, and helped by the things discovered during the analysis.

Those who practise narco-analysis aver that, even if it brings to light no more than analysis in the waking state, it has the virtue of being much quicker, and allows the detection in one or two short sessions of material which psycho-

---

1. *Transference* is 'a phenomenon by which the patient projects onto the person of the doctor the symbols of his unconscious needs, so investing the physician with a peculiar authority' (Cornil and Ollivier, *Etudes de neuro-psycho-pathologie infantile*, p. 42).

2. Cornil and Ollivier, *op. cit.*, p. 7.

3. Or *should* follow: only too often the patient whose mind has been so to speak 'taken to pieces' is left with these pieces and is given no help in building them into a new and truer pattern.—*Tr.*

analysis would take weeks or months to reach. This is because it so rapidly allows an increase of affective contact, gives the patient confidence in the doctor, and brings about the transference which is an essential aspect of the treatment. It further enables one, by using carefully measured doses of the drug, to graduate also the 'dose' of consciousness allowed to each patient during the treatment session.

It is doubtless too early to draw up a balance sheet of the complex matters in which startling successes can be set against equally obvious failures. Here, however, are the main lines on which the results can be assessed, according as narco-analysis is envisaged as a means of investigation of criminal responsibility, of diagnosis, or of treatment.

On the first point, it is certain that pentothal removes the ability of consciousness to deceive, and brings to light thoughts which, though consciously known, are deliberately concealed. In this way its use helps one to fix on an emotional incident which has either been deeply repressed or which has been masked by fear, and which is the focal point of many neurotic symptoms. On the other hand, it is very doubtful whether analysis under pentothal brings real unconscious material to the surface, and equally certain that it does not reach the deeper-seated complexes.

Narco-analysis is a means of reaching a diagnosis by collating all the psychological and somatic manifestations which it brings about. It is also useful in this field because some cases produce psychopathic reactions relating to latent syndromes, and therefore helps the classification of doubtful cases. It helps, for instance, to differentiate between hysteria and true epilepsy, the hysterical fit being precipitated under narcosis. In stuporose cases, it may help to differentiate melancholia from paranoia in its form of 'persecution mania'. It may also bring to light a latent and exaggerated sense of guilt, while in the psychopathology of children it differentiates superficial difficulties from constitutional perversions.

In the field of therapy the results are less certain, yet one fact seems to be established, which is the good results on neurotic symptoms arising from *recent* emotional shock. This applies especially to such cases as those of war neurosis, which were numerous, and, as already stated, it was American army psychiatrists who advanced the case for pentothal most effectively, especially as, since the war, complete cures, free from relapse, have been reported. This type of neurosis is caused by memories which are associated with emotional shock and charged with an abnormal amount of feeling. Consequently, whether deliberately and consciously, or involuntarily and unconsciously, they become repressed by fear and horror. This leads to a kind of unconscious stagnation which upsets the balance of the personality, and fills it with anxiety. Pentothal here acts in two ways.

In the hypnogogic state it removes all conscious refusal to remember. It also soothes the anxiety which involuntarily erects a carrier preventing the return of some memories and the discharge of their abnormal emotional content. After this has happened, they can be restored to their normal place in the memory of the patient, as part of his conscious mind.

But beyond these simple cases, nothing is certain. There are a few reports of improvement in deep and long-standing neurosis. But where psychosis is concerned, if pentothal at times allows an exploration of the mind in mild cases, it is important either to investigate or help the treatment of any deep mental deterioration or disintegration of the personality.

Together with these results it is necessary to consider the dangers of narco-analysis. These arise from the fact that the patient narcotized with pentothal is exceedingly suggestible. This is aggravated by the fact that, as often as not, the patient does not speak spontaneously, but has to be

PSYCHIATRIC ASPECTS

questioned. This clearly requires great delicacy of touch, great finesse and care on the doctor's side. He has to ask questions, yet he has to try and be an entirely objective witness of the answers given. Moreover, he must endeavour to keep to a minimum the number of drug sessions, else the patient may lose faith. He must avoid leading questions which may suggest to the patient ideas which complicate or aggravate his trouble. He has, moreover, to try and avoid too violent an 'abreaction', such as might cause serious results and even lead to suicide. Narco-analysis, in short, adds to the dangers of the Freudian system those of hypnotic suggestion. There is a risk of facilitating certain dangerous delirium-like reactions. One must beware of trying, in this tricky situation, to do anything which might create the very thing one is trying to cure.

All practitioners, it is true, do not agree on this point. But even those who do not think that suggestibility is increased admit the possibility of a distortion of the psychic organism.

> One cannot let oneself forget that the *whole* organism, and the brain in particular, are affected by a toxic drug. There is consequently no doubt whatever that the psychic picture is seen only through the prism of a barbiturate.

There is therefore no reason for believing that narcosis will produce a statement of factual truth:

> The fact that during narcosis the power to pretend and to deceive are inhibited, paralysed, or, on the contrary made obvious, does not mean that the revelation of secret wishes or deep attitudes of mind are always the expression of factual realities.[1]

The task of interpreting what is revealed is thus considerable. Narco-analysis *'must never confine itself merely to a passive registering of the psychological material shown by the patient'*. Otherwise the risk of mistakes is great, and the practitioner naturally has to avoid them. Professor Delay

---

1. Cornil and Ollivier, *op. cit.*, pp. 11, 40.

tries to broaden the field by correlating psychological analysis, with its many uncertainties, with an analysis of bodily behaviour, gesture, mimicry, posture.

It must be admitted that there are many cases where, even with a good technique and careful preparation, results are mediocre, partial or non-existent. This is why one must always add to psychic exploration the observation of bodily phenomena which pretty certainly give positive information in every case, and much instructive material.

Yet even with the data thus weeded out, this 'psychosomatic' narco-analysis is a highly tricky thing.

The interpretation of the data obtained from chemically induced psycho-analysis must be passed through a very fine sieve of criticism. The method requires great experience and deep psychological knowledge. . . . These are essentials if narco-analysis is to keep any real value and not become a danger in the hands of incompetent and inexperienced physicians, and particularly that it should not fall into the realm of romance and purely fantastic interpretation.[1]

It is only fair to add that most practitioners are not only cautious where the technique of narco-analysis is concerned, but also as to the morality of it. There is nothing which requires more care than this more or less enforced confidence, and as one of them puts it in a neat phrase, it can only be legitimate within the framework of 'a moral contract'[2] between patient and physician, a framework based on trust and free acceptance—outside of which contract narcosis would only be an encroachment and a violation. Moreover, it should be essential to prepare the patient in advance to give his trust in such a way that it will still be there after the treatment. It would be both unethical

1. Cornil and Ollivier: *Problèmes de sélection et d'actualités Médico-sociales*, pp. 145–146.
2. Cornil and Ollivier: *Etudes de neuro-psycho-pathologie infantile*, p. 40.

and insufficient to try and bring this about solely by reliance on the effects of the drug. One cannot speak too highly of the deep solicitude and the kind of fraternal compassion which redouble the wariness of the investigator and which alone can justify the use of such a drastic procedure.

It would, of course, be wrong to think that all psychiatrists are agreed on the efficacy and beneficial results of narco-analysis. Naturally enough, the negatives are not often exposed in scientific journals, where it is more usual to report success rather than failure. But in private talk more doubts are allowed to show through.

> Certainly [writes one practitioner] I have had positive results, but only among patients whose mental illness was, according to usual clinical prognostications, likely to improve anyway. They would, however, have taken longer. I have also had spectacular results with a sudden lifting of inhibition, but these have been followed by relapses, and sometimes by a state worse than the first.

And again:

> As with all new techniques, one hears at first a flood of favourable comment. This is soon followed by a few critical articles, the number of which increases until finally it is seen that only a few cases really benefit from the new method.

This, of course, is one of the features of all research. Let us not forget how medicine has its own passing fashions. Who, for instance, still uses the methods of hypnotic suggestion exactly as practised by Charcot? Who uses Freudian analysis in its original form and without any kind of reservations?

There is not even agreement on the exact scope of the method. Some psychiatrists try to bring about complete cures under narco-analysis, others, afraid of bringing about further distortion, new defence mechanisms or of encouraging an insidious form of drug addiction, use it only at long intervals and even perhaps on a single occasion. The first consider narcosis as a therapeutic system, the latter use it only to clarify and orientate themselves in dealing with difficult cases. There are a third class which allow nothing in its favour, having found that it gives them nothing they did not already know or could not find out by using only the classical method.

From these differing views we can draw no conclusions either for or against the purely medical use of narco-analysis. This is neither within my competence, nor is it my purpose. But it was right to give evidence both as to the narrow field and the uncertainty of the procedure. It would be scientifically dishonest to pretend that a method in which research is still only feeling its way, is so well founded that it should be uncritically allowed to enter the field of judicial enquiry. It is quite certain already that there is no justification for suggesting that narco-analysis is a technique for interrogation and forcing confession. Moreover, there is no ground for insisting that a method about which psychiatrists are at once so cautious and so divided among themselves can even give certainty as to the amount of malingering or of criminal responsibility. And narco-analysis is not so rich in results that one should be too definite in asserting that it has any value even in a straightforward expert diagnosis for legal purposes.

In short, there is neither enough certainty nor, for that matter, is there any need, for this method to be used outside the clinic, and in a Court of Law. We shall discuss later both the legal and the moral reasons why such a transfer should not take place. At this point, let us confine ourselves to the statement that there is no scientific reason for urging positive action towards using it, for it is science itself—the very doubts of scientists—which set a limit to the legitimate use of narco-analysis.

2. AMPHETAMINE SHOCK

The use of amphetamine shock in forensic medicine has not yet been explicitly discussed. It is nevertheless relevant to our purpose to give some medical data on this new method.[1]

Let us remind ourselves that the procedure consists in the intravenous injection of a massive dose (15 mgm.) of methyl-amphetamine. It is a shock method, one of violent dislocation of the psychic organism. In this it is akin to all such methods: electrical convulsion shock, insulin shock, cardiazol shock. The principle involved is the same: either the sudden lifting of inhibition or the penetration of amnesia, so that morbid elements can be discharged. In short, it brings about a disintegration of the psyche so as to allow its reorganization on a new pattern.[2]

Amphetamine shock has only a very limited therapeutic use, and its principal value seems to be only in diagnosis,[3] and that only in the psycho-neuroses.

In neurasthenic depression, the action of methyl-amphetamine is spectacular. It is obviously not a radical cure, but its value lies in its temporary effect, especially if it should make psycho-therapy possible.

In moderate doses and over a long period it gives a certain feeling of euphoria which may help the psychotherapist in

1. Delay, etc.: *Le choc amphétaminique* (*loc. cit.*, p. 309). Justin-Besançon: *Les psychamines* (Entretiens de Bichat, 1948). Sabrie: *Nouveau développement dans l'étude des amines psychotomiques* (Revue Médicale française, 1948). *Annales Médico-psychologiques, passim* and especially, 1947, pp. 50, 271; 1948, p. 80.

2. I have, on occasion, suggested that these shock treatments are comparable to taking a bottle of boiled sweets of which the contents had stuck together, and banging it on the table. The sweets come apart, their arrangement after the shock may be different, but the contents of the bottle remain the same, and tend eventually once more to stick together. The analogy is not perfect: sometimes the bottle breaks, at other times, perhaps, the morbid pattern is broken by the discharge (abreaction) of emotion. But the results justify the comparison—unless, of course, active psychotherapy can be and is used to bring about a real change in the contents and not only the arrangement of the mental 'bottles'.—*Tr.*

3. All that follows is from Delay, etc., *Le choc amphétaminique* (pp. 315 *et seq.*).

the treatment of chronic neuroses and in depression consequent on infectious diseases. Apart from that, and especially where there is disintegration of the personality (i.e. in psychosis), amphetamine shock has nothing but diagnostic value. '*It has absolutely no therapeutic effect*', but, by letting loose or by accentuating in dramatic and brutal fashion some of the patient's symptoms, it may clinch a diagnosis. In short, one makes a person already mad, more mad, in order to be sure that he really is mad, and with what kind of madness.

Here is how Professor Delay classifies things. It is in maniacal states that amphetamine shock is most dramatic.

> The syndrome is always temporarily aggravated, whether this be by pressing hypomania into full mania, or by increasing mania already in evidence, with frantic motor activity, and a spate of words quite incomprehensible because it comes so fast.

In melancholia one has the same spectacular increase of symptoms. The shock aggravates anxiety so much that it occasionally shows itself in a paroxysm of fear causing a wish to commit murder or suicide, so that it has to be antidoted at once with barbiturates. It is especially in the stuporose forms of melancholia that the shock is instructive, because it breaks through the mutism which prevents investigation, and brings fantasies to light, especially those of guilt and self-accusation.

In schizophrenia, where there is disintegration of personality, amphetamine shock has more complicated results and allows a deeper differential diagnosis to be made. Catatonic tendencies are aggravated, and all the more so if they were masked prior to the injection, the patient showing the wax-figure immobility or the typical slow-moving agitation, going through a series of stereotyped and repetitive movements, or tending to remain in any position in which the body is put by the physician. On the other hand, loquacity is less and may even become mutism. Where there is no catatonia, the shock may either bring it on or clarify the schizophrenic picture by emphasizing the discord and ambivalence (contradictory words and actions), fantasy, disorganization of speech (inventing new words or phrases, etc.), which help one to make an early diagnosis in doubtful cases.

It is interesting to compare the reports on amphetamine shock and those on narco-analysis.

There are cases where the barbiturates have no effect, but amphetamine allows investigation and perhaps makes therapy possible. Latent anxiety, for instance, which pentothal would further stifle, is activated and made visible by amphetamine. The same applies where barbiturates fail to bring about emotional discharge and amphetamine does.

It seems that the two methods have different indications. Narco-analysis exposes the unconscious, and its field lies in the exploration of hysterical amnesia, while amphetamine shock, by forcing a momentary objectivization of consciousness acts more on conscious or semi-conscious reticence and reservations.

There are some cases in which both methods link up. One may use barbiturate narcosis to attenuate the results of amphetamine shock as soon as the diagnosis is established, and especially to check anxiety if it shows signs of getting out of hand. In the reverse direction, one may use amphetamine shock after a preliminary narcosis to increase the discharge of emotion by bringing the narcosis to a sudden end, thus causing explosive liberation of latent and unconscious material.

Gradual narcosis with amytal, followed by hurried awakening with metedrine makes verbal externalization of the contents of consciousness so urgent that it has an explosive force hitherto unknown.[1]

Here, too, my aim is not to criticize the medical value of these dreadful methods—which are, anyway, in their

1. Delay: *La narco-analyse ne doit pas devenir le sérum de vérité* (*Figaro*, 12 Nov. 1948).

infancy. But in view of their brutality it is impossible not to feel qualms of anxiety should they overflow the limits of purely psychiatric use. Nobody has yet, to my knowledge, suggested their use in legal cases.[1] Doubtless it is because such procedure for bringing about mental disintegration causes some fear even among their promoters, and even within the narrow field of medical therapeutic practice, let alone outside it. Yet there is no security if it once goes beyond the walls of laboratory and clinic.

The medico-legal problem is the one that principally concerns us, so we shall concentrate our study on the use of barbiturates for narcosis in criminal cases. In this connection we must never forget that pentothal is only a beginning and that the whole matter is growing and becoming more serious. Narco-analysis and amphetamine shock are inter-connected. How then can one consider the use of one in judicial procedure without thinking also of the other? If pentothal should, for good reasons, be refused admission to the Law Courts, these reasons are strengthened by the appearance of the fearful companion which stands by its side.

[1]. Which does not exclude the fact that they may have been used in practice. We shall quote later on a case where pervitine was used in a diagnosis of malingering.

Chapter 3

THE MEDICO-LEGAL ASPECTS: FROM MEDICINE TO POLICE METHODS

THE medico-legal problems connected with narcosis now have to be considered, and that with the greatest care and exactitude. I myself believe in the need for absolute and unequivocal opposition to it. Yet this opposition, to be effective, must be accurately aimed or it will miss the mark altogether. It is a complex, if not a subtle, question, but in that complexity the force of my protest must not be allowed to become obscured. It would be useless to raise at once a loud outcry about police tortures, we must first tackle the matter on the very grounds, and in the same terms as the partisans of pentothal. The discussion of these will need serious attention. I apologize, but anything glib and superficial would be both vain and risky.

1. DIAGNOSIS OR EXTORTION?

The most spectacular effect of pentothal, and that which has been most disingenuously placed before the public, is the inhibition of voluntary control of the mind. It can thus, we are told, show up a malingerer in that if a person refuses to speak, or denies things, or pretends not to remember, pentothal narcosis makes him confess the motives which prompt this negative attitude. By removing conscious resistance to interrogation, pentothal offers the police the temptation of using it as an easy method of bringing about a confession.

By presenting things in this light it has been possible to impress on the public the current expression 'truth serum', implying that pentothal makes the liar tell the truth. A formula at once simple, untrue, redolent of 'Americanism', and one which quite distorts the whole matter.

It is nonsense anyway: pentothal is not a serum, and, as to truth, it is a word rashly applied, since, as we have seen, whatever comes out of such interrogation under narcosis has little in common with factual reality. The subject is sometimes refractory and continues to watch his words, at other times he is over-suggestible, when it becomes necessary to interpret what he says with the greatest caution. The truth is *not* spoken openly, hence there is great risk of it being more than necessarily obscured.

If then it should have happened that certain police forces have used pentothal as a means of extracting confessions, French physicians and jurists have, on the contrary, resolutely refused to allow the question to be considered only on that level. They will not use pentothal as a truth serum because they do not mean to act as inquisitors or executioners, and they have no illusions as to the veracity likely to be found in a confession under narcosis. That is doubtless why one of the experts mixed up in the Cens case said several times, '*The truth serum is humbug. It does not exist*,' thus suggesting that no practitioner has ever believed in it, nor expected pentothal to be used as a means of causing confessions to be made, nor that the accuracy of such a confession should be taken for granted.

The problem of pentothal as it stands to-day is therefore not that of its use in police interrogation, it is that of its use in forming expert medico-legal opinion. It is then an extension of straight psychiatry, though obviously not as a matter of *treatment*, but as one of *diagnosis*. The medical expert is charged with informing the judge as to how far the accused is responsible for his acts. This is his only duty, and, far from using pentothal narcosis to obtain a confession, he may use it only to assess how much the pathological elements in the subject's mind relieve him of responsibility, and how much control he could have exercised over what he did.

THE MEDICO-LEGAL ASPECTS

It is in these terms that the matter was brought before the Medico-legal Society (of France) in a communication from Professor Delay.[1]

In the cases of two accused people, detained because of mental trouble, pentothal was tried experimentally and with therapeutic intention, not for forensic purposes. In the first, an aggressive attitude towards the victim of the crime was exposed. This had hitherto been concealed. In the second case it showed a form of deception which was not entirely deliberate, as it overlay and was dependent on a genuine mental disease-condition. The narcosis thus brought to light both a quasi-voluntary amnesia and the beginning of disintegration of the personality.

The interest of these experiments lay in that it made it appear as if pentothal were able to furnish the data required for medico-legal diagnosis and determining the relative responsibility of the person accused of a particular crime. Let me add that the test, far from being pushed on towards attempting to obtain positive admission, showed, on the contrary, the limits of its effectiveness on this point, as both the subjects remained on the defensive. The first, when asked, 'Who did the killing?' answered, 'There are some things one cannot tell.' The other said, 'I can remember when it suits me. When it does not, my memory fails me.' It thus became simply a matter of diagnosis, not of extortion. The authors of the paper explicitly stated that the method used, capable as it was of '*determining the pathological mental condition and what voluntary factors were super-added ... cannot pretend to assess the value of confession to a breach of law: which, anyway, would be contrary to the principles of justice actually in force.*' The problem was thus very exactly stated to the Society.

This body then appointed a commission charged with framing a resolution. After discussion in which there was

---

[1] Delay, etc.: *Intérêt Médico-légal de la narco-analyse* (*Annales de méd. légale*, No. 4, April–May–June 1945, p. 55, pub. Baillière).

much discord, hesitation and vacillation, the commission proposed the following:

> The Medico-legal Society (of France) resolves, that the use of methods of investigating the unconsciousness such as pharmaco-dynamic explorations under pentothal should, in principle, be approved in medico-legal expert assessments as a purely medical matter and as a means of diagnosis. But the medical expert cannot feel confident that the revelations obtained under the influence of the drug on the actual facts of the case are exact. In this way the determination of criminal responsibility shall never be made on this test alone, the interpretation of which demands a critical analysis on the part of the medical expert. In any case, it is recommended that the method should only be used after the failure of all ordinary methods of investigation.[1]

This shows that the approval given to narco-analysis in legal cases is qualified by many reservations: i.e. it may be used as a means of diagnosis, but not to obtain a confession, and if a revelation of guilt is received, it is subject to the seal of medical secrecy. Moreover it can only be used after the failure of other means.

This amounts to saying that pentothal should be used in law only as a means of expert medical assessment, not as a means of forcing an avowal of guilt.

This resolution, despite its many reservations, was not accepted by the Society. Even before it had been discussed, a formal yet vigorous objection was raised by the Association of those physicians who had been deported or interned for political reasons during the Resistance. At its meeting of 8 December 1945, this association charged two of its members, Professors Charles Richet and Henri Desoille (the latter himself an official of the Medico-legal Society), to draw up a statement of which the following extracts give the salient points.[2]

---

1. *Annales de méd. légale*, No. 6, Nov.–Dec. 1945, pp. 178 *et seq*.
2. Richet and Desoille: *A propos du procès-verbal* (*Annales de méd. légale*. Jan.–Feb. 1946, p. 27).

THE MEDICO-LEGAL ASPECTS

Those making the protest began by pointing out the risk of a misuse of the procedure of narco-analysis and the abuses which might result from this.

We protest with all our strength against this resolution. We protest in the name of our comrades who fought for the respect of individual freedom and who underwent interrogation by methods they found objectionable. To pass such a resolution opens up a path dangerous from every point of view. It is not permissible to use chemical methods to deprive an accused person of his free will—that is, of one whom French law presumes to be innocent (until proved otherwise).... We cannot agree to it also because we are afraid that this violation of mental integrity may lead in the future to abuses. At any time the method might be used as a convenience and the restrictions on its application be forgotten. Interrogation by this means may become a part of police procedure. One might, for instance, use it to obtain an avowal of political views. We know only too well the abuses which come when coercive methods are used in interrogation, to agree that the honourable principles of French law should be changed in this way.

The protest goes on to point out that medical secrecy as to any information obtained by expert witnesses could not properly be observed:

The expert witness would have to delete from his report both the symptoms observed and any discussion of their meaning. He would have simply to express his own opinion. The resolution proposed is inadmissible, for an expert's report must be complete and sincere, since both the defence and the prosecution have the right to argue about the conclusions reached by him. They can only do this if the observations leading to that conclusion are an integral part of the report submitted.

A third paragraph insists on the distinction which must be made between the legitimate use of pentothal in psychiatry and its improper use in forensic matters:

These new methods ... must only be used therapeutically. When, after far-reaching changes, our penal system comes to consider some offenders, not as guilty people needing punishment, but as sick people needing care, then only will it be right to use pharmaco-dynamic methods to explore the unconscious. The diagnosis will then be the first step in therapy and will have only medical repercussions. In the proposition before us this is not so, for if the first aim of diagnosis is to decide whether or not punishment should be meted out, it may have repressive results.

The Annals of the Medico-legal Society apparently show that it dropped the matter. It had no further public discussion of the question and in this way tacitly refused to proceed with the resolution.

True, it may not always be wise to draw conclusions from silence, but in this case there is reason for doing so. I do not, of course, suggest that the matter is as finally disposed of as if a clearly negative formula had been accepted. But it is plain that the present attitude of the Society is something more than a mere abstention from expressing an opinion, one which might be taken as giving consent to the method. Silence coming after a proposition agreeing to its use, countered by formal opposition, implies something much stronger and more positive. It would be wrong to believe that the Medico-legal Society, under whatever reservations, would tolerate the use of pentothal in criminology. It has, at the very least, *refused* to authorize it, and in the light of the terms of the protest which stopped the proceedings we have the right to believe that it has actually and quite definitely condemned it, in view of present conditions. One must thus hold the opinion that any medico-legal expert assessment performed under pentothal contravenes not only the usages and customs of judicial procedure in France, but also the feeling of the body of medico-legal opinion in general ; and that, even if it were to be carried out within the framework of the rejected resolution. It would be untrue to say that pentothal tests, even if medical secrecy is respected, are in line with the position adopted by the

Medico-legal Society. What *is* true is that this body refused to adopt a proposition which authorized the use of pentothal at all, under any such circumstances, and no expert can claim to be working with its permission.[1]

It is nevertheless obvious that the question is not settled. Polemics still go on, opinion is split, and the Cens case has not made matters easier. The problem in any case is intricate. If it was a matter of choosing between extortion of confession on the one hand and respect for free will on the other, the debate would be closed, for among jurists or physicians there are none who agree to the rape of a person's conscience. The point at issue is the legitimacy even of a diagnosis made under narcosis.

Has the Richet-Desoille protest failed to go to the heart of the matter, since its primary objection is to the use of pentothal in interrogation? This procedure was, it may be said, already rejected by medico-legal experts, and if so, the act of laying the matter before the Medico-legal Society leaves things where they were and no conclusions can be drawn from it.

I think otherwise. The very terms of the protest give us grounds for continuing the debate because they show that there is no clear distinction between extortion and diagnosis, and that inevitable deterioration would allow the medical method to degenerate into something like a police procedure.

2. THE PROCESS OF DETERIORATION

If we consider the first paragraph of the protest, it does indeed reach the core of the matter despite the fact that it does so indirectly. It is important that we should see what is the basic purpose which inspired it.

It is that in this kind of affair it is less vital to consider the actual procedure, and more so to see the abuses which

[1]. Which is quite the opposite of what was stated in *Le Monde* (25 Dec. 1947), and in an article by Dr. J. Declos, *Narco-analyse* (*Sciences et avenir*, Feb. 1948).

it may lead to, to condemn it in principle because one anticipates the harm which may result from it. Maybe my opinion is due to blind obstinacy, but I propose to cling to it and I can support myself by quoting many other examples where delicate procedures have been used only under the greatest safeguards, yet where there has been the risk of these safeguards being abrogated when convenient.

We live in a barbarous age, a time when people are apt to overlook subtleties and the strict limits to action which such subtleties demand. Moreover, there is a weakening of the respect man should have for man, and scientific techniques are used in order to degrade others. There is a slippery slope between forensic medicine and police torture, and it becomes essential to check the descent. When one is menaced by barbarians, one does not throw open the gates of the city.

Whether one likes it or not, there lies the problem. There is no purpose in theorizing on the value or morality of the principle underlying medico-legal use of narcosis, and nobody will doubt the theoretical difference between a medical diagnosis and a forced confession. But there are subtleties which are likely to disappear when it comes to practical matters. That is the essence of it all: it is deeds which count, and one must constantly hold before the partisans of the use in law of narco-analysis the question, 'What will grow out of the method once it becomes current usage? Will not policemen soon allow themselves to misuse it to extract admissions? And are you so sure both of your technique and of yourselves that you can guarantee that the exact mark between medicine and police practice will never be crossed? We do not doubt your good intentions and we know that you have said that this method should *never* be used by the police, that it *can* never become part of police procedure.[1] These statements promise nothing but your own good will, your own belief—which may be naïve

---

1. Divry and Bobon (*Acta med. leg. et soc.*, p. 644), Ollivier, *ibid.*, p. 642. Delay, *loc. cit.* (*Figaro*, 12 Nov. 1948).

or perhaps arrogant—in the security provided by your privileged position. You set a good example, but others, less scrupulous, may not follow it. When people who are policemen at heart, but who have obtained a few diplomas, use your precedent as authority, who will then be able to attack as illegal their use of this kind of medicine?'

That is the crux of the matter, and the Richet-Desoille resolution was not mistaken. It is not they, but those who persist in discussing and justifying the use of pentothal on theoretical grounds, who are evading the real issue.

Can it be said that all these fears are of things which may never happen and are irrelevant? If so, we must pass on to the second point of the protest to show that the restrictions and precautions advocated for the use of pentothal are already proved ineffective, for it is in the very nature and action of the method that the danger lies.

It seems from the somewhat involved terms of the proposition laid before the Medico-legal Society that reliance should not be placed on the factual aspect of any confession. Moreover, no analysis of these should be made in Court to justify the expert's conclusions, so as not to weight the evidence in either direction. Those who protested against the original proposition wonder that it has not been realized that a report in these restricted times is useless, since both prosecution and defence have the right to discuss it. Such a report, they say, must be both honest and complete. If so, how can professional secrecy as to confessions be kept? The medical expert, assuming he obtains a confession at all, is on the horns of a dilemma: is he to give a full report, when he may be guilty of having forced an admission of guilt, or is he to make it only partial and so valueless?

This matter was discussed at length at the International Academy of Forensic and Social Medicine.[1] The report of

1. At an International Congress held in Liège in 1947. The report, by Divry and Bobon (*Acta med. leg. et. soc.*, Brussels, April 1948, pp. 601–655), has already been quoted.

this carries all the more weight from being subtly and scrupulously fair as well as because it was drawn up by a practitioner entirely in favour of narco-analysis.

True, the expert witness does not have to report every detail and can omit material irrelevant to the mental condition of the subject. For instance, suppose, in a matter unconcerned with his wife, a man confesses to unfaithfulness: this has nothing to do with the question of responsibility for a criminal act.

The report says that *'one may receive confessions which may be interesting in shedding light on our religion, but which are not essential to the establishment of a medico-legal diagnosis'*. But the expert is not a recording machine, his job is to discriminate and analyse. His conclusions are not articles of faith either to prosecution or defence, and the Court has both the need and the right to know how the subject has 'shed light on' the said 'religion'.

There is a third kind of confession, that having strict bearing on the crime with which the accused is charged. Here those making the report distinguish two cases. Most of the time, they say, the admissions obtained tend to diminish the degree of responsibility, at any rate in the eyes of professional justices expert in interpreting the evidence— but, unfortunately, not in those of a 'lay' and often incompetent jury, which may moreover be prejudiced, and may make its decision only on the superficial appearances of the confession.

In the second case, where the confession may have bad repercussions on the accused, the medical expert cannot fail to see the incompatibility of the purely medical aspects of his case with the requirements of a fair defence. For the confession has not been obtained spontaneously, and it may truly be held that it was made under duress and should not be heard in evidence unless freely repeated by the accused, in full consciousness and under normal conditions. The expert witness may thus find himself trapped in a highly unpleasant position.

Against this, it is useless to say that narcosis practically never causes confessions. We shall see later that this is untrue, for the trust which is evoked by the very fact of the questioner being a physician may lead to his receiving admissions. But they are confessions of quite another nature than those of actual criminal guilt, a point we shall refer to later.

The very nature of the process of narco-analysis and the conditions defining its use are thus likely to take the expert into an untenable and ambiguous position, where medicine and police methods are inextricably confused. What then is left of the theoretical distinction between diagnosis and extortion? It is lost even in the most cautious use of the method, let alone when it is used improperly.

This may indeed be thought to be a purely technical matter. But it is much more than this because it is redoubled by moral and ethical consideration. Narco-analysis is a specialized method of mental investigation depending on the *surrender* of the individual. And to use it under conditions where this surrender—which is almost impossible under normal conditions and at the will of the patient—is obtained by force or by cunning becomes, however well intentioned the operator, morally unjustified.

All psychiatric technique, whether for diagnosis or cure, rests on trust between physician and patient. This belongs in essence to every medical situation, as without it this situation loses its truly human character. It is particularly important in psychological medicine, where the very soul of the patient has to be exposed and opened up to view. Whatever faults Freudian psycho-analysis may have, it is entirely right in emphasizing that the psychiatrist must assume and deserve the rôle of confidant. It would be wrong to think that any technique involving the use of drugs absolves him from this, and in narco-analysis the surrender of the subject which follows the use of the drug should be freely agreed to *before* the drug is used to bring it about, as well as freely given *afterwards*, as the cure goes on. This is an essential guarantee of the 'humanity' of the method as well as its possible medical efficacy. It is only fair here to draw attention to the scrupulous care with which some practitioners of narco-analysis try first of all to create this relationship of confidence. Even in this instance, morality comes first, technique after.[1]

The relationship between medico-legal expert and accused are almost the exact opposite of those between patient and doctor. No doubt many experts do not see the situation as a duel, but place themselves also in the position of helper and protector. Yet even if the two are not antagonists, there must necessarily be suspicion on both sides: the first suspects the other of trying to evade him and wants to tear down his mask, the second fears that the first is not his well-wisher and so prepares to defend himself. What can be the outcome?

Let us however suppose, if only to cover the whole ground, that trust has been given, and that the accused, freely and without constraint, agrees to surrender himself to the doctor. There is no fault to find with this, except that it is to the expert's credit. But he is then entrusted also with the task of reconciling in his professional conscience the conflict between the medical and the forensic aspects of his duty. Conscience should here be paramount, since confidence has been given simply on the plane of ethics and not because a particular technique is being used.

If on the other hand confidence in the doctor has arisen only under or after the actual narcosis, the medical expert's situation is quite different, and he should refuse to accept it in the way he may if it is freely given. '*Why*,' says one writer,[2] '*should one not use pentothal for fear of receiving admissions of guilt, since one also gets them without it?*' There is clearly no moral or judicial analogy between confessions obtained by these means and those obtained by

1. Cornil and Ollivier, *op. cit.*, pp. 16, 40.
2. Trillot: *Utilité de la narco-analyse en méd. légale* (*Acta med. leg, et soc.*, p. 651).

freely given trust. Narco-analysis brings on only an *enforced confidence*: two words which are incompatible. This applies even if the subject has agreed to the use of pentothal, for it does not follow that he realizes, or clearly appreciates, the possible effects of the injection, that it may lead either immediately or as an aftermath to his losing his power to keep silent or to speak only of certain things and not of others.

What then is the situation of the expert? If the material he lays bare helps him to find extenuating factors and to diminish the guilt and criminal responsibility, all is well, not only for the accused but also for the doctor, who has acted in the proper rôle of a physician rather than a prosecuting counsel. And even if the prison system refuses as yet to accept his contention, he will at least have declared that the prisoner is a patient in need of therapy rather than a wicked person needing punishment. The relationship of trust is thus preserved and sanctified *a posteriori* and by its aftereffects even if it was not so *a priori*, by the intentions of the doctor to heal rather than help to punish.

On the other hand if the confessions made under narcosis force him to state that the prisoner is indeed responsible for his actions, the expert is to be pitied for the equivocal situation in which he has landed himself. If he feels the full weight of responsibility with which this enforced confession loads him, how can he escape from the sense that he must preserve medical secrecy? It is indeed a paradoxical situation for an expert witness to feel constrained to suppress part of his evidence! But if he rejects the moral bond, there is no situation in which he is more blatantly and flagrantly guilty of breach of confidence—a double breach since it was first obtained without free consent, and then because it is used to bring about punishment. This is not merely a technical difficulty, it is a straight matter of morals.

Professors Ollivier and Cornil have made a suggestion which, despite its prudence and reservations, seems to me inadmissible for similar reasons. They say that one might justifiably suggest narcosis to the accused: if he accepts, it is an indication of his innocence, if not, it would presume his conscious responsibility for his acts.[1] But, even assuming the highly doubtful proposition that pentothal will, indeed, make innocence evident, the advocates of medico-legal narco-analysis are still among a tangle of contradictions. For it is obviously illogical to offer a suspect the right to refuse if, by using that right, he adds to the belief in his guilt. The duress is less obvious and more insidious: it becomes a form of blackmail. But if he accepts, then why give the injection? It is obviously useless and morally unjustified since this very acceptance means a giving of medical confidence which should gag the physician. At the same time, if the doctor does not give it after it has been agreed to, he is guilty of having played a trick on the victim. One is then really more deeply embedded in the tangle around the very police methods one has tried to avoid.

To preserve the dignity of the medical profession, and for the medico-legal expert not to degenerate into a police auxiliary, it is necessary to adhere strictly to the limits drawn in the Richet-Desoille protest: that is, the use of pentothal only as a medical technique, not as a judicial method. Never must the demarcation between its use as a diagnostic and therapeutic measure and its use as a means of crime detection be allowed to become obscured.

There is still worse to come. We have already seen that every reservation, restriction and precaution which can be placed round the use of pentothal, and the very distinction between diagnosis and a forced confession vanish when it is used for medico-legal purposes.

Let us remember that it was proposed to the Medico-

---

1. *Problèmes de sélection et d'actualités médico-sociales*, loc. cit., pp. 150–151.

The same idea is suggested by others, such as Trillot, in *La narcose barbiturique en médecine légale* (*Annales de méd. lég.*, July–Aug. 1949, p. 170). It is only fair to add that Prof. Cornil has, much to his credit, revised his views on the matter.

THE MEDICO-LEGAL ASPECTS

legal Society that pentothal should be employed only for strictly medical purposes. This in itself is ambiguous, since the only purely medical act is that done for therapeutic aims. In expert medico-legal assessment this is not so. We may allow that the intention of those framing the resolution was to differentiate between diagnosis and extortion. Yet even this is disregarded when one expert says that narcosis '*should be applied without restriction wherever there is even the slightest suspicion of deceit or malingering*'.[1] And, more explicitly,

> it is not essential that the terms of reference of the doctor should formerly charge him to unmask deception: the duty of every psychiatric expert making a deep mental investigation *ipso facto* implies the unmasking of deceit. It is evident to us that if the accused has the right to lie and to prevaricate, the examining psychiatrist has not only the right but the duty to make certain that he is lying, and to prove that he is pretending.[2]

This clearly advocates the use of pentothal in an entirely non-medical rôle, and simply as a 'lie-detector'. I shall exemplify this shortly with an example where a traitor to his country pretended to be insane. Every means was used to unmask him;[3] cardiazol convulsions, repeated narcoanalysis, and even pervitine given under false pretences, with an untrue statement as to the effects of the drug. The victim held his ground, yet the expert's report resulted in a sentence to death. Granted we were dealing with a real deceiver. But can this merciless battle, this pursuit to the death, possibly be called a *medical* act? Here already is a precedent to any future abuses which arise in the attempt to outwit the deceiver.

The resolution had a second clause, by which the expert was told that he must not rely on the things disclosed being

1. Divry and Bobon, *op. cit.*, p. 630.
2. Divry and Bobon, *op. cit.*, p. 627.
3. Divry and Bobon, *op. cit.*, p. 636. '*Everything is good which can bring out the truth,*' says another expert. '*The expert has the duty to use any means in his power,*' says another.

factually true. This too goes by the board when, though the details of a confession are passed over admissions in general terms are allowed even if obtained as a result of such a hunt after deception. This too is clearly agreed to by another expert,[1] who writes:

> The day may come when physicians will be called in by the police or the prosecuting officers to apply narco-analysis for the purpose of obtaining confessions from all accused people.

I do not believe this. I believe rather that the police themselves will operate—perhaps with the connivance of some renegade practitioners, while one hopes that the judiciary itself will never stoop so low. This quotation suggests neither more nor less than the revival of the rôle of inquisitor from of old. And despite the fact that the writer recommends that this operation shall be entrusted only to physicians who are '*competent, conscientious and who are deeply versed in the method and aware of its fallibility*', it is easy to see how lightly these precautions would weigh when once the fundamental principle is accepted, that pentothal is a proper drug to use in police interrogation.

The third reservation is equally void. It was recommended that the method should be used only after ordinary procedure has failed. Where is the precise limit, and by what objective standard can this failure be measured? In the Cens case, the line was crossed at once—and this was a case where classical methods had already given a clear and conclusive diagnosis.

In short, nothing remains of all the attempts of some experts to maintain a distinction between diagnosis and extortion, such distinction being effaced by the experts themselves.

Yet a further threat is added to our uncertainties as to the kind of use which might be made of pentothal. That is the tendency of some who wish to use it in all and every case.

1. Trillot, *op. cit.*, p. 653.

Some, it is true, want to keep it only for exceptional instances. But one legal expert, Professor Lebret,[1] thinks that it is easy to work on the basis of a direct opposition between the strictly medical use of narcosis and its use in criminal investigation. The problems arise in many cases midway between the medical and the corrective level, for instance where preventive detention is in question—i.e. not exactly punishment, yet detention coming within the framework of the law rather than of strait medicine. These present themselves in three layers going from the more medical to the more punitive:

(1) In deciding to continue or to finish the detention of a patient in a mental hospital. (2) In attempting to re-educate minor delinquents. (3) Whether or not to keep accused people in custody when their mental state is in doubt. After this we come to purely punitive measures, these in turn being at two levels; (4) in matters of probationary liberation and (5) for examination prior to any decision as to detention.

This is an excellent classification, provided that the multiplication of intermediate steps should not in effect abolish these steps and lead to the use of pentothal in all stages on the excuse that the movement from one stage to the next is imperceptible and cannot be defined. The argument is, briefly, that if narcosis is useful in making apparently pure medical decisions, yet such as lead to deprivation of freedom, why refuse to allow its use in more directly punitive cases? The slide-over is particularly easy in the reasons given for passing from 4 to 5. For one may easily agree with periodical medical examinations of cases to be released on ticket-of-leave, and admit that narcosis is

---

1. J. Lebret, professor of Law at Aix, *Sur la licéité du recours à la narco-analyse*. (Report made to the Congress on social and legal medicine, Lausanne, 1948, and published in *Annales de méd. légale*, March–April 1949, p. 58.) I refer also to a letter in which Professor Lebret told me of this report before it was published. I want to express my thanks to him, despite the strong opposition I feel to his ideas.

legitimate and harmless because it is negative and may set a person free or that, at worst, it may advise continuation of a detention already in existence. But if one may use narcosis in order to get a person free from prison, there seems little reason for not using it also to put him into gaol .

I do not think that Professor Lebret could have done better than argue this way, had he intended to show the dangers ensuing from the use of pentothal in criminal law.

In any case, Professor Lebret's plea rests on the supposition that the prison system is already capable of dealing with cases from a therapeutic as well as from a penitential angle. This is open to doubt. In advocating the use of pentothal both in endeavouring to liberate and to imprison, he is working on a hypothesis of the indeterminacy of such imprisonment. *'The judicial procedure (by which the term of imprisonment is set) is not a much more serious matter than the decision made some years later as to the ending or continuation of such imprisonment.'* This might clearly lead to serious abuses, and, as the author himself recognizes, penology has not yet reached the point required, and to introduce pentothal in the present state of things is indeed to put the cart before the horse.

Professor Lebret realizes the delicacy of his position and uses all his subtlety and knowledge to show the legitimacy of the use of narcosis. For if it is to be used as a means of cross-examination it should take place in the presence of both judge and counsel. This is out of the question, of course. The physician would object, even if the others should be willing to be present. Yet, he argues, there are exceptional cases in which counsel for the defence may be absent during an examination, and it might be in such cases that narcosis should be introduced. The argument goes on to show that both technically and legally *'this would not be a formal interrogation'*, only *'a particularly subtle investigation of the mind'* of the accused. Which is merely sticking a different label on the same thing. The dangers are obvious.

Yet another writer[1] suggests a general use of narcosis in order to show up malingering, particularly (1) among soldiers who try and escape from their patriotic duties, especially in time of war, and (2) in the realm of pensions and social insurance, where, to avoid exploitation of the State or of private insurance companies, the expert has, it is suggested, the right to use harmless but efficient procedures to bring the truth into evidence.

Clearly, the advocates of pentothal mean to see that civic virtue, the safety of the Motherland and the interest of the State will be most vigilantly secured. The next thing will be that somebody will propose the use of narcosis to combat tax evasion!

There is even an element of comedy in some of the pleas brought forward. We have already mentioned a German physician who proposed to hypnotize witnesses. The idea of the resulting perfect witness thus handled by the experts, made honest by technical means, has always haunted the dreams of some. We have a passing but interesting sign of this in the report of the committee of the Medico-legal Society.[2] One of its members drew attention to the fact of the capital importance of expert assessment of witnesses. (In practice, of course, it would simply mean that witnesses would flee whenever possible, and refuse to come forward unless made to.) But, pentothal being the main subject under consideration, another member, misapprehending the line of thought of his colleague, hastened to say that witnesses must be spared narcosis. We seem to have had a narrow escape! But clearly, the idea is in the minds of people, and who can say where we shall stop? Perhaps somebody will one day suggest that both counsels, and even the judge himself, should be dosed with pentothal before the trial. And, as a final step, it might even happen

1. Trillot: *La narcose barbiturique en médecine légale*. Communication made to the Congress of Legal Medicine, Lausanne, 1948 (*Annales de méd. lég.*, July–Aug. 1949, pp. 168–170).
2. *Annales de méd. lég.*, No. 6, Nov.–Dec. 1945.

that somebody will advocate that the whole trial take place in the light of truth revealed when all parties are, at the time itself, under the influence of the drug!

To sum up: the partisans of pentothal flatter themselves that they can keep the use of pentothal in law strictly to matters of diagnosis. I think, on the contrary, that it is inevitable that the medical procedure must become prostituted when it is used in police cases. Man is still too much of a barbarian to be trusted with it. Further, the 'truths' revealed are of a dubious character. The expert who uses pentothal in legal cases finds himself caught in a moral dilemma. And the declaration of its advocates and the practices of some, speak for themselves.

It is on account of the certain moral deterioration which must take place, which, indeed, is already taking place, that we find the basic reason for prohibiting altogether the use of pentothal in legal procedure.

CHAPTER 4

THE CENS CASE

[This chapter is a condensed version of the original. The French text goes into many details of legal procedure which do not apply to this country and which, without the proper background, have little significance to the British reader. Hence I have tried to present the facts of the case as clearly and concisely as possible, but only to suggest the principles involved and without changing the spirit of the author or, I hope, omitting anything relevant to the general argument.—*Tr.*]

IN December 1947, while only medical circles were as yet discussing the use of narco-analysis, a famous case drew the attention of the public to the question. The Press aggravated things by using sensational reports, but in any case the feelings roused were a sign of the healthy spirit still to be found among the French people. Opinion has now cooled off, and this makes it easier to obtain an objective assessment of the facts, basing this on the evidence and the documents of the case. These show the undoubted fact that there was a very grave miscarriage, both of justice and of medicine.

THE FACTS

Henri Cens was born in 1919 and entered the regular army in 1940. When, after the capitulation of France, the army was disbanded, he joined the North African Police and was stationed at Tunis, where he served under a Superintendent called Marty. The latter was transferred in 1944 to Toulouse, where his collaboration with the Germans in trying to repress the Resistance made him notorious. It may be that the association of Cens with Marty, though this ended long before the Toulouse atrocities, prejudiced his case: Cens never served under him in Toulouse, having been sent to Montpellier before Marty's own transfer to this town. In 1943, during a prison riot in Montpellier, Cens was accidentally wounded by a revolver bullet which entered the left fronto-parietal region. He was operated on the same day and the bullet was removed, but he thereafter suffered from right-sided hemiplegia and complete aphasia.

In November 1945, he was arrested on a warrant of the Military Court of Algiers and taken to the hospital of Fresnes Prison, near Paris. Every medical examination confirmed the diagnosis already made. A Doctor Paul called for an immediate neuro-psychiatric report as to whether Cens was in a fit state to plead, and even to be detained in gaol. In December, Dr. Génil-Perrin stated that his transfer to Algiers was inadvisable, and that the aphasia made him quite unable to explain himself or to speak in his own defence. He added that he thought there might be slow improvement by re-education. He thought the patient fit to remain in the prison infirmary, but recommended his transfer to the annexe at Nanterre for special treatment.

No notice was taken of this recommendation, despite the fact that Cens' condition was deteriorating, with serious and frequent attacks of Jacksonian epilepsy. Many further certificates were issued until, in January 1946, Dr. Thouvenel, the prison medical officer, insisted that, in view of the aggravation of the patient's condition, it was impossible to move him from Fresnes to Toulouse, where, in the interim, the papers relating to the case had been transferred from Algiers. Moreover, he emphasized the need either for special care at Nanterre, or else his release from prison on medical grounds. Dr. Thouvenel was met with such supreme indifference from the Public Prosecutor that he protested openly and said that such behaviour was unworthy of a country which pretended to be civilized. Meanwhile, Maître Murat, who became counsel for Cens

THE CENS CASE

in May 1946, being unable to find out from Cens himself why he was in prison, had to enquire from the prosecution as to the nature of the charge against him. In September 1946, in the face of renewed demands for his transfer to Toulouse, and despite the number of statements that this was impossible, Maître Murat demanded an expert examination at Cens' expense to try and settle the matter once and for all.

Three experts, Doctors Génil-Perrin, Heuyer and Laignel-Lavastine were instructed in October by the examining magistrate of the Court of the Seine *Departement*. Their reports, sent in in December 1946, confirmed the existence of clinical signs which made malingering out of the question and proved him unfit to be moved or to plead. They went further and said that he was incurable and even deteriorating by reason of the fits, and recommended medical discharge.

The inertia of the judiciary went on. Maître Murat put in several requests for liberation during the year 1947, and never even received a reply. He then applied to the War Ministry and to the Keeper of the Seals for the case to be removed from Toulouse, which had no reason whatever for dealing with it, to the Court of the Seine. Silence continued to reign, and at the end of 1947 Cens was still in prison.

Despite all the statements that he was not fit for the journey, he was moved to Toulouse in January 1948. Meanwhile, the examining magistrate had instructed the same three experts to re-examine Cens. The terms of this instruction spoke of the 'many and grave accusations': a matter of no concern to the doctors, and which might only prejudice them against the prisoner. They were also—despite all previous opinions—asked once more to state their view as to his fitness to plead, and also as to his need for special treatment. This insistence acquired the air of an invitation to the doctors to contradict their earlier statements so as to justify *a posteriori* the prolonged detention.

A new report was sent in in October 1947, which drastically changed the original one. The organic troubles were admitted, but, while the first saw the aphasia as a direct consequence of the injury, the second, though the clinical signs were precisely the same, concluded that Cens *could* answer questions, that the aphasia was nearly cured, and that if there were any recurrence of speech defect, this was pure malingering.

Why was this? Because one of the experts used pentothal narcosis on Cens, telling him it was *for therapeutic purposes*, and hence obtaining his consent. As Cens came back to consciousness, he uttered the one word, '*Oui*', which was taken to prove that his aphasia was incomplete. It should be noted, of course, that between the two reports, he had been undergoing re-educative treatment, and a few days later he was able to explain to the doctors that for eight months he had been training himself to speak. But he was afraid that the judge would think he was malingering if he spoke badly, so he had decided it was best to say nothing at all. This may seem to justify the report that Cens was now much better in this particular at least, but a subsequent report (see below) shows that the diagnosis of malingering was quite unfounded. As to the epilepsy, the first report accepted the straight evidence of nurses and co-prisoners, the second said the fits were simulated, on the grounds that he had one while recovering from the narcosis, and this was not typically Jacksonian. Moreover, when the gardenal (luminal) which he had been having to control the fits was stopped, neither the severity nor the number of attacks increased.

The report concluded, (1) that Cens was entirely responsible for his acts, when he was wounded—a fact nobody had questioned; and (2) that he was paralysed but was not, or was no longer, aphasic, hence that he was fit to plead; (3) that he was fit to be detained in prison. The last two points are in direct contradiction of the first report by the same experts. It was on this, and despite the fact that neither magistrate nor medical experts expressed an opinion on the matter of transfer, that Cens was moved to Toulouse under conditions of the greatest moral and physical distress.

It was through an indiscretion that the newspapers had their attention drawn to the case in the first instance, but the more important sequel took place in the Courts. Maître Murat here drew attention to the extraordinary new method which had been used, and to the fact that it was contrary to the traditions of justice, of respect for the accused, and to the rights of the defence. He also pointed out other irregularities on points of law. Among other things, he showed that Cens had been questioned on his arrival in Toulouse without his lawyer being present. He emphasized not only the contradictions in the experts' reports, but also that use had been made in them of the results of an operation which had been agreed to only as therapeutic, not forensic, so that the right of the individual had been grossly infringed. Thus, in February 1948 the general problem had already been clearly stated: that the accused must be left by the prosecution in full possession of his faculties, and that it may use no form of violence, direct or indirect, to deprive him of his free will. In the Cens case this principle had been grievously infringed.

While this was going on, the Council of the Order of Barristers ordered Maître de Coulhac-Mazérieux to report on the whole question of the medico-legal use of narco-analysis. This report, presented in July 1948, emphasized certain essential points such as the inviolability of the human person, whether free, suspect, or in prison; his right to be safeguarded against invasion of the privacy of his own mind and spirit by any form of attack, and especially against those means which would diminish his self-control. Moreover, the accused was declared to be entitled to refuse anything which would assist in convicting himself, and so has the right to be silent and even, if he wishes, to try and deceive. The value of a confession made under any form of constraint is nil, while the expert, instructed by the judge, disposes of no more freedom in the use of force than the judge himself. A resolution was then passed by the Council, which is an unequivocal condemnation of the use of pentothal in justice, and the Chairman was charged with passing on this decision to the knowledge of the Public Prosecutor.

Cens was meanwhile taken to Toulouse and in May 1948 he was once more submitted to expert examination by Doctors Lafarge, Perret and Gayral. The conclusions of these once more categorically contradicted the controversial second report from Paris, while confirming all the previous ones. It made the question of the aphasia even more precise by saying that the trouble was not so much one of ability to articulate as of the ability to fit words to the ideas in the patient's mind: which accounts for the improvement which had taken place by re-education, as also for relapses under conditions of fatigue or anxiety. In short, the genuine nature of the physical symptoms was confirmed. A month later, in June, Doctors Riser, Noguès and Trillot examined him once more, and again the earlier diagnoses were confirmed, a fit of *petit mal* being noted while the patient did not know he was under observation—and hence unlikely to have been simulated in order to impress anybody. It was further noted that the patient was a very emotional man, that the physical symptoms would be aggravated by this, but that there was no evidence whatever of attempted malingering or deception.

By now, too, re-education of speech had helped so much that Cens was deemed fit to plead and to answer questions. This report, the last of many, was made in November, after several visits to the patient. A few days later, on the only occasion when any promptness was shown in the whole lamentable affair, the Toulouse Court adjourned the case *sine die* and released Cens on medical grounds. He had now been in prison three years, and that in a state of health which, from the first, entitled him, under French law, to be set free.

The case was prolonged by a civil suit brought against the experts Génil-Perrin, Heuyer and Laignel-Lavastine, on the grounds that the worst wrongs done to Cens arose from the use of pentothal—i.e. a year's extension of imprisonment, as well as the transfer to Toulouse and the refusal of proper treatment; besides which he had been deprived of the comfort of a weekly visit from his wife and children who lived in Paris. He claimed substantial damages, as well as charging them with assault on the person by means of an injection to which he had not agreed, and which was not compatible with normal legal procedure. He further complained of violation of medical secrecy, since it had been alleged that the narcosis was being used as treatment, not as a means of obtaining evidence for legal purposes.

Cens was allowed legal aid in this suit. The Press was ironical about a needle prick being called a wound, and about medical experts being bound to secrecy. The medical profession itself was divided and there was not the usual closing of the ranks in defence of a colleague, though a number of articles written by high authorities implied enough to confuse the issue in the public mind. The first day of the hearing in Court became a matter of medical and forensic discussion in which the experts, by their defence of themselves also defended the use of pentothal. The gravity of the principle became obscured by the personal issues.

On the second day, in February 1949, Dr. Heuyer conducted his own defence, not wanting, he said, to embarrass any barrister by asking him to plead in defence of a practice just condemned by the Bar Council. He spoke brilliantly, carried the day and was discharged. Yet, as we shall see later, careful examination of his own statements condemn the method he was trying to defend.

The case ended when Cens' petition was dismissed on 23 February 1949. But the judgment equally dismissed a cross-petition of the defendants. Not one of the whole areopagus of professors, physicians and lawyers said a word to show that they were conscious of the deeper spiritual aspects of the whole matter.

A point which arose was that narcosis had been used with therapeutic intent. This raises the further question whether there can be any therapy for malingering: i.e. for lying by action rather than by word, or else pretending to be in a psychopathic state which would prove lack of responsibility for any crime committed. Obviously, one cannot *cure* malingering, which is not a disease, one can only show it up. Doctor Heuyer's report confuses the issue when he speaks at once of therapy and of the intention to unmask malingering, and it shows a prior prejudice towards thinking the aphasia suspect.

If malingering were an illness, it could be treated: but then the word would lose all judicial significance. If it is not an illness but a wilfully chosen state, then Cens, a sick man, was no malingerer, since his disease was unequivocally organic, and tallied with his injuries. Moreover, both his attempts at re-education, and his frank statement to the doctors as to his fear of upsetting the judges, tend to bear this out. Nothing in his behaviour suggests in any way that he tried to use his illness to deceive and so escape his just due.

The whole assessment of the case as one of malingering, turning on the one word, 'Yes', said during narcosis, followed subsequently by his explanation of his mutism even after much effective treatment, is belied by a straight and unchallengeable diagnosis based on his physical disabilities. Moreover, the narcosis was used under false pretences, medical secrecy was violated, and to make matters worse, the diagnosis of malingering was accepted by the Court.

The judgment given on 23 February 1949, in the suit against the experts, also repays examination. It accepts the fact that an injection was given for purposes of medical expertise, but deems that this is not,

1. an assault, even slight, on the person, because it was given,

   (a) for medical reasons, to make a diagnosis. Moreover, Cens was a malingerer and the diagnosis sought to unmask his malingering. (Both of these statements are false.)

   (b) for legal purposes. In this there was no assault because Cens consented to the injection and, moreover, the prick of the needle caused no pain. Yet even if it were true that psychic integrity and freewill were infringed, there is no law to impose sanctions on that account. (What then is an assault? And, moreover, it is clear that there is a deficiency in the law.)

2. a breach of medical secrecy. The Law asserts that the expert must tell the judge everything. (Which, as we shall see, makes the position of the expert using illegitimate means of extracting information quite untenable.)

The whole judgment is highly regrettable, as it seems to endorse the use of methods which infringe the privacy of the conscience of the individual. It is said that Cens agreed, lay down, presented his arm for the injection. But it is also evident that Dr. Heuyer misled him as to what the injection would do. It is clear that the consent of the victim should only have been asked for after explicit explanations of what was involved.

Another point was that of malingering, diagnosed only at this particular examination, and negatived at every other. Had Cens been really a malingerer, he would have been badly placed to bring such a suit. If not, he had a just claim for reparations. Yet, in defiance of the evidence, he was called a malingerer and denied damages. It is further clear that the distinction between *the physician treating a patient* (as was averred by Dr. Heuyer in his statement as to why he gave the injection) and of the *medical expert acting on judicial instructions*, was confused and obscured. The whole affair was a scandalous miscarriage of justice, not on one point but many.

Discussions among jurists grew out of the case. They centred on the refusal of the Court to qualify the experts' actions as assault, especially as, Cens not having (as is usual and correct in medical practice) first solicited their help on his own account, they intervened on the orders of the judge and so were in no sense physicians in the course of the usual practice of their art. Hence the act of giving the injection was in a different frame of reference from that of doctor and patient.

One commentator concludes

> The judgment can in no way be approved. On the contrary, it seems extremely regrettable and vexatious that the archives of French jurisprudence should contain a decision declaring that it is legitimate to use scientific means to suppress the freewill of an accused person, and so allow the prosecution to enforce its will—that is, in plain French, to use violence on him.

The Cens case is clearly an outstanding case of principle, quite apart from the stir it caused in French public opinion. It raises both forensic and medical problems, and it is to be regretted that the plaintiff did not appeal against the decision of the Court. That he did not do so is however intelligible: he is a very sick man who only wants to be left in peace. Nevertheless, the charges against him are not disposed of despite the indefinite adjournment of his trial. Yet, an informal appeal has resulted and judgment has been given: the medical profession have learned caution and their opinion is divided; learned societies are moved. And, despite the actual result of the case, it has become morally impossible for an expert to use pentothal in such a case. The Cens case has killed it.

The basic principle however remains to be clarified. It has been argued that a single case proves nothing and that one mistake should not condemn the whole method. But this one instance has shown up much wider problems: those of the true principles of justice; of the position of the scientific expert; of the value or otherwise of certain techniques of narco-analysis, both in law and medicine; and above all, the inalienable spiritual and moral rights of the individual, even if he is accused and guilty of crimes whether against a person or the State.

Chapter 5

FORENSIC PRINCIPLES: JUSTICE *VERSUS* TECHNIQUE

THE use of pentothal in legal cases issues a challenge to the very position of the medico-legal expert. This makes it imperative that we consider the exact conditions under which he has to work.

'The work of the medical expert is limited by the terms of a finite assignment,'[1] says Faustin Hélie. Unless the expert is wise enough to keep strictly within these terms he may feel tempted to go beyond the limits of his juridical function, to allow himself autonomy and to make claims which are contrary to the principles of real justice.

1. THE EXPERT'S MANDATE

The criminal code says nothing specific about the reports made by specialists and experts of all kinds, nor as to the means to be used by them in carrying out their task. From this one may conclude that he has the right to employ all the means which 'science' places at his disposal. That is, when it comes to medical matters, that every method of investigation and diagnosis may be deemed legal which helps him to draw conclusions and to assist the judge.

Yet it is obvious that such latitude must have limits. It is on this that experts differ. They are certainly unanimous in eliminating anything savouring of physical violence or causing danger which the penal code might call assault or

---

1. 'L'expertise n'est qu'une mission.' The French phrase cannot be exactly translated.—*Tr.*

grievous bodily harm. But even apart from this elementary principle there is much divergence of opinion. The boldest think it would be a pity if the expert were not allowed to use 'modern methods of investigation'. Others think he should keep to methods already well tried and established. Yet even here some would allow such things as lumbar puncture, electro-encephalography, the taking of blood specimens and other physical acts which, though in a minor way, infringe the physical integrity of the patient. Others refuse to go beyond simple interrogation and commonplace clinical examination of pulse and reflexes, and the use of the stethoscope.[1]

Scientific arguments alone cannot decide the matter, since the application of the term *science* itself is in some doubt. It is in the name of scientific progress that it is urged that new and still untried methods be introduced into forensic medicine, and that despite the fact that science itself demands that no system should be used as if it had made its proofs until such proofs have indeed been given. The concept of what is scientific is too fluid to enable us to say exactly when the required degree of certainty has been obtained, and we must therefore look elsewhere if we wish to decide what is justified in expert examination.

We shall find it illuminating to see why the Law is silent about the details of expert examination. No doubt it is because it is only recently that the Bench has had recourse to expert scientific opinion. As science progressed, moreover, a tradition gradually and quietly grew up of what such experts could decently do and not do. There has therefore been no need to make specific rules as to what is allowable, because they are the very same as those of the code proper to the examining counsel or magistrate.

The expert has no independent function. Instructed by the judge, he should use the means proper to his speciality in the same spirit as that judge, and with the same respect for the fundamental principles of criminal procedure. What

1. *Annales de méd. lég.*, Nov.–Dec. 1945, pp. 178 *et seq.*

the code lays down for one applies equally to the other, and its silence on the special rôle of the expert implies that the function of the expert must be identified with that of the judge.

It is thus in the light of the legal theory of the *mandate*[1] or assignment that we have to interpret the silence of the legal code. We shall see that it is in fact much more restrictive than permissive, and that the expert who wishes to use his mandate as authority to employ '*every means*', to '*set everything to work*',[2] would be committing a grave mistake.

The expert is instructed by the judge or magistrate who obviously cannot delegate to another powers he himself has not got. Hence the expert has no more authority than the judge, and what is forbidden to one is also forbidden to the other.

That the fields of authority are identical does not, of course, mean that identical methods must be used. If a judge instructs an expert, it is so that the latter should make use of the methods peculiar to his branch of science, but only provided he is guided by the same principles as to what is required and allowed in drawing up an indictment. It is thus in terms of jurisprudence, not of science, since science has not helped us, that we shall have to discriminate what means may be used in expert assessment. We shall have to know, not only whether it is the most suitable, the most up-to-date and the most efficacious, we must also ask ourselves whether it is in line with the general spirit of our code of Law, and more especially with that relating to criminal cases.

1. Attorney-general Tahon: *La liberté individuelle et un nouveau procédé d'expertise mentale* (Address at the opening of the Appeal Court, Liège. Reported in the *Journal des Tribuneaux*, Brussels, 26 Oct. 1947). De Coulhac-Mazérieux, *op. cit.* (*Gazette du Palais*, July 1948).

2. 'When the magistrate instructs the expert to find out whether or not the accused is responsible, the expert must set everything to work to obtain clear and accurate answers' (Dr. Charlin, *op. cit.*, p. 166).

'Every means are justified,' says Dr. Heuyer. Divry and Bobon hope that 'every technique for psycho-somatic investigation may be used.'

This theme is argued by a jurist,[1] who suggests that the expert's task is simply to perform an act of *technique and medicine*, and not one of law. But it is not a purely technical act since it has a forensic purpose and becomes part of the process of determining criminal responsibility. And if, as he says, the expert merely gives an opinion which the judges need not accept, that surely is an additional reason for considering his work as subordinated to legal authority, not as an autonomous action.

The expert's task is thus to fulfil an assignment, by his own methods, but for the purposes laid down for him by others. The principle is clear enough, but because it is not appreciated many experts become confused as to their rights and their duties.

One of the points at issue is how much right the expert has to put pressure or constraint on an unwilling suspect. The first mistake, made even by one of the committee appointed by the Medico-legal Society, is to obscure the very clear question of criminal procedure, '*Has a suspect the right to refuse to be examined and questioned by an expert ?*' and to drown it in the more indefinite question as to the right of the medical man to intervene and force treatment on a patient whose illness is dangerous to others. This, of course, trenches on a still wider field, and discussion would become endless, as to the respective rights of the individual and of society. But even if a solution were to be found on these lines, it would not really advance matters, for if the law gave the physician the power to *treat* a guilty person whether or not he agreed, it would still not cover the case of the *expert witness*, as against the physician, and his right to force a certain mode of investigation on a suspected criminal, against his will. Only a consideration of the authority given to the judge can guide us. The judge cannot force the accused to speak, though he may draw certain conclusions from his silence. The latter may therefore also

1. Robert Vouin: *L'emploi de la narco-analyse en médecine légale* (Recueil Dalloz, 16 June 1949, pp. 106 *et seq.*).

be deemed to have the right to refuse to submit to special investigations, and all the expert can do is to register that refusal and perhaps to express his opinion on its significance. It is for the judge to interpret matters, taking into account the whole of the evidence in the case.

If anything beyond this is allowed, many difficulties are to be foreseen. Some experts already quoted wish to use narco-analysis wherever they think fit, and even against the will of the patient. This would mean the passing of a law backed by penal sanctions in case of refusal, similar to that which authorizes the police to photograph and measure a person under detention. Such a law might, however, have bad repercussions in that it would absolve police or expert witness from being charged with assault were he to use coercion on a recalcitrant prisoner. Moreover, how would such a threat help? It would merely be an additional argument to the blackmail, '*If you refuse, you add to our suspicions of you.*' This is entirely contrary to the spirit of justice. For what can be the value of examining a suspect threatened with sanctions if he chooses to say nothing? He would be in an impasse: punished if he speaks, punished also if he does not. We should be going back to the '*infamous tormenting of truth*', of which Voltaire spoke in connection with the oath forced on the accused when being questioned under torture.

Not to contravene the principles of our laws, the partisans of constraint may suggest that it be applied only in specific cases, selected by the highest judicial authorities. But, apart from the fact that it is physically impossible to give an injection, carefully dosed and timed, to a resisting patient, what then would be the result? It would take a platoon of orderlies to hold him down, and even then, '*what would be the reactions produced by fear, anger, despair? And what accidents might not occur, quite apart from an infamous and undignified spectacle, unworthy of the name of justice?*' —or of medicine.[1]

1. Tahon, *op. cit.*

The mistake made by these imperious experts is to think that legal authorities have the right to handle prisoners exactly as they please. One[1] thinks that the examining magistrate[2] may order a medical examination '*under the threat of physical compulsion*', and that, if the accused person '*does not usually object, it is because he knows that the magistrate has discretionary powers and would not hesitate, in case of need, to have him forcibly carried into the consulting-room.*' The writer agrees that even there, the victim might still resist, in which case, the intravenous injection '*would be almost impossible and the doctor would give up attempting it so as not to assault the patient.*' This is a strange idea: that force should be used only to lead in the end to the abandonment of force. It is anyway most unlikely that any judge or magistrate would lend himself to such futility, even if his sense of the spirit in which he has to perform his task did not already deter him. For the discretion of which he disposes is not an absolute power: he may decide that certain expert examinations are necessary, but he cannot force a recalcitrant prisoner to submit to them. If the prisoner refuses, his task is to note and record the fact. The expert has no greater authority than this.

On the second point, that of unmasking deception, we have already shown the confusion likely to arise in the medical sphere. Further misunderstanding on the position of the expert may arise as to this from the legal angle.

Some experts declare with enthusiasm that the revelation of deceit is a natural, and perhaps a chief part of their task. It would be in fact an encroachment on the judge's work. We are told that '*every deep investigation of the mind* ipso facto *involves the unmasking of deceit*'.[3] This may be true from the medical viewpoint, where the diagnosis of a mental state must cover both the pathological factors and the

1. Logre: *Narco-analyse et médecine légale* (*Le Monde*, 30 Nov. 1948).
2. *Juge d'instruction:* see footnote 3, p. 23.
3. Divry and Bobon, *op. cit.*, p. 627.

voluntary elements. But from that of the Law the expert has no *automatic* right to draw a conclusion of voluntary deception and moral responsibility. The old school of medico-legal experts was wise when it held that their task was to make scientific enquiry into the mental state of the subject, holding that the determination of responsibility and intention was not a medical matter, but belonged to the judge's province.

True, the judge may want to know whether the subject's mental integrity is such that he can answer questions, and the expert should give a scientifically determined reply. But he is going beyond his duty if he speaks of *voluntary* deception, as this is a question of morals, not of medicine. To think that the judge can ask the expert, '*Is the suspect a malingerer?*'[1] is pure imagination. I have so far no evidence that any judge has ever asked such a question otherwise than indirectly, by implications underlying the dialogue between him and the expert. This seems to have happened in the Cens case. But to ask a direct question would be for the judge to renounce his particular function and to ask his agent to make a judicial pronouncement which is outside his competence. It follows that the experts who insist that their task is to detect lying are in effect usurping the function of the judge.

This notion of the extension of the expert's duty supplies a pretext for taking on himself the privilege of using methods which would not be allowed to a judge. This has been clearly demonstrated by those advocates of narcosis who claim the right to use every technique for psycho-somatic investigation, without restriction as to method. This is doubtful medical ethics and, moreover, a forensic monstrosity. If the accused has the right to lie to the judge but not to the medical expert, this is an invitation to the judge to pass accused people over to the expert, who could then freely employ constraint. The result would be not justice but a caricature.

1. Logre, *op. cit.*

FORENSIC PRINCIPLES 87

In short, arising out of the claims of some experts, we have a series of misconceptions. These focus round one most significant statement made by one already quoted, '*I believe that every method is permissible which enables us to find out the truth.*' The expert here claims to seek for truth: this is the judge's province, not his. He claims the right to use *all* methods: the judge is not allowed to do so. In fact the expert places himself in the position of judge but without the restrictions which hedge round the judge's prerogative. In short, he tries to make himself at once doubly omnipotent, yet to remain free of responsibility. The dangers are only too clear.

2. JUDICIAL EXAMINATION

A person accused of a crime is really submitted to interrogation at two levels. The first is by the police, whose natural bias is to obtain a confession of guilt. Hence (after, in Britain, the suspect has been cautioned that anything he says may be used in evidence against him), the function of the police is—like that of the prosecuting counsel—to try and outwit the subject, to trip him up, to entangle him in contradictory statements. In the hands of an unscrupulous police system, this might obviously lead to abuses and to an indiscriminate use of any form of pressure which will bring about an admission of guilt.

Examination in Court, however, is different. Even though the function of the prosecution is much the same as that of the police, this is met by the defence, whose task is to attempt to cancel out the arguments advanced from the other side. The purpose of the procedure is to try and preserve an innocent person from being punished for crimes he has not committed. Moreover, in civilized society it is deemed preferable to let the guilty go unpunished rather than run the risk of persecuting one who is not. For if the criminal code is aimed against the wrong-doer, the rules of justice and trial are aimed at doing no harm to the honest man; whence the presumption of innocence until guilt has been proved.

Fair play is guaranteed in the rules which insist that the accused must know the exact charge against him, and those which warn him that he need answer no questions until his defending lawyers are present; in the freedom to choose those defenders, and so on. There is also the general spirit which guides the judge in his choice of the exact procedure to be applied in any given case.[1] It is incumbent on the expert to observe this spirit, and determines the attitude which should be taken towards narco-analysis.

If a person is to be deemed innocent until found otherwise, no procedures should be applied to him which one would regret having used if his innocence is eventually proved. He must be treated as a free person, able to decide for himself how much or how little he is prepared to answer questions. Between examiner and accused there should be a man-to-man relationship which effectively forbids any form of constraint.

Clearly, therefore, direct physical violence, blows or torture are absolutely forbidden; so is indirect violence such as prolonged interrogation, prevention of sleep, starvation, fatigue from bright lights. But moral violence is also excluded, and this means anything which deprives the subject of his freedom of mind, or lessens his power to choose whether to speak or keep silence. All jurists are not agreed as to the exact point where constraint begins, but they are all inclined to firmness rather than leniency.

It would be absurd to denounce all form of questioning, on the grounds that even if properly conducted it submits the accused to some degree of pressure and makes him feel hunted. This would mean that the case for the prosecution would have to rest entirely on objective proof of the facts

---

1. That is, in Britain, such things as remand for medical examination, for reports from various experts, the use of probation, etc.—*Tr*.

FORENSIC PRINCIPLES

of the case, and without reference to any statement made by the one accused.

On the other hand, one must respect the integrity of those who are actuated only by the highest motives of justice and truth, and who therefore object to anything which savours of trickery, deceit or subterfuge in the way questions are asked. For such, true justice can only use truth in its enquiries, and any deception or attempt to mislead the prisoner degrades the examining magistrate to the rank of police inquisitor.[1]

That on which everybody agrees, and even those who admit that the examining officer may use dialectic skill and art, is to proscribe all form of cheating or trickery, or the setting of traps with which to nullify the freewill of the accused. Such methods may redound to the glory of a policeman, but would compromise the dignity of any judge or magistrate. This point was decided in January 1888, in the Court of Appeal (in France), sitting as the Supreme Council of the Magistracy. An examining magistrate had been brought before it because he had telephoned to a man believed to be an accomplice of a suspect released on bail. The magistrate pretended to be the accused, and thus obtained by fraud proof of the guilt of both parties. This was a fine catch, no doubt, but the case was taken away from the magistrate and he was severely censured for his action.

These matters concern only indirect methods of tricking the subject out of his freedom of choice—actually, surprising rather than nullifying it. What then of methods which attack it directly? We have already mentioned the affair of the anonymous letters in Tulle, in which the magistrate was dismissed for attempting hypnotism on the suspect.

Thus, apart from all doubts as to the psychological and scientific value of narco-analysis, it is clear that from the legal point of view it is as inadmissible as hypnosis. Both of them interfere with the mental freedom of the individual

---

1. See Faustin Hélie: *Traité de l'instruction criminelle*, 1866, vol. IV, p. 579.

and infringe that which is the most precious and inalienable possession of man.

3. THE PARAMOUNT RÔLE OF LEGAL PRINCIPLES

Expert investigation by means of pentothal, while being, as we have seen, contrary to the principles behind the drawing up of a case, can go further, and in fact upset the whole judicial process. Once more, it is the theory of the systematic unveiling of deceit which confuses matters.

It was to be hoped that the reservations, slight though they might be, placed around the suggestion that pentothal should be used in law might have defined the limits of the expert's field. They showed a desire to make his report a part of the evidence presented to the Court, and not to give it a determining place in the general process of trial for crime. But, by a bastard theory, part medical, part forensic, the expert is led to believe it to be his duty to expose lies.

Let us imagine a suspect, up to a certain point silent, amnesic, or simply denying the charge, brought back before his accusers with an expert's report that he is a liar. This diagnosis would be obtained not by the careful consideration of ordinary clinical signs, but on narcosis, for which all the prestige and weight of modern science is claimed. Such a report must influence the examining magistrate so profoundly that it may be said that the interrogation is made useless and is already concluded. For whereas the magistrate might previously have had certain suspicions and hence the right to shape his questions accordingly, he is now confronted with an alleged scientific certainty which gives him no latitude in interpreting the answers given by the accused. No ordinary questioning is, under these circumstances, either possible or useful: the suspect is lying and that is all there is to it. Hence he must be guilty, nobody can believe his statements or protestations, his very silence becomes an admission of guilt. The expert's report becomes a verdict of 'Guilty' and leads to condemnation.

FORENSIC PRINCIPLES 91

The defence is also paralysed, for what can it do with a client already convicted as a liar? The lawyer is an auxiliary to justice and has to serve both higher interests and those of his client. His rôle is only possible where, even in the worst of cases, there is some chance that justice may be tempered by extenuating circumstances and facts. But this possibility is absent when everything the accused may say becomes automatically vitiated by his supposedly known intention to deceive. Can defending counsel co-operate with a client who has been unequivocally and scientifically proved a liar? If so, he would be helping to defeat the ends of justice.

The accused cannot even gain anything by pleading guilty, for any excuses he may make for his conduct would be looked upon as further insincerity.

How, too, could a judge reach a verdict based on his true inner convictions? There would be no hope of the defence helping or influencing him in any way, no hope that the judge would be able to transform that verdict by considering fine shades of meaning. We should, in short, be returning, under the mask of science, to the system by which, once guilt was proved, the judge had no discretion to assess the degree of responsibility, but would have to give a sentence based on a tariff fixed according to the particular offence. In short, the verdict would be made by the expert, sentence would automatically follow. The examination prior to trial would be reduced to an injection, the defence to silence, and the judge to recording the expert's conclusions. What would remain of justice? Nothing but a rigid form of determinism, without any of the liberty given by a judgment based on appreciation of grades of responsibility. In short, a pseudo-scientific caricature of equity.

The foregoing shows how ineffective the restrictions suggested would be when once narcosis began to be used. And, far from placing the expert in his proper rôle, it would lead to his acquiring a vastly exaggerated authority, all the more so if, because of the rules of medical secrecy, he were to be allowed to affix the label 'intentional deceiver' without having to explain why he did so. Prosecution and defence would have to argue their case in terms of whatever detailed evidence they could bring forward, the expert would not. The judge would have to listen to the arguments of both sides and sum up openly and in public, the expert need only say one word, without being called upon to justify it, shielding himself behind the plea of medical secrecy. *'The expert would then become a kind of judge from whose ruling there was no appeal, and who could pass his verdict without explaining the reasons for it.'*[1] Indeed a paradox: the Law, obliged to justify its actions, would allow science to act arbitrarily and to keep silence about its own doings. This would be the inevitable result of allowing the *imperialism of the expert:* a medico-legal dictatorship, which would deprive the Law of its superiority in its own sphere over claims made on the plea that they belong to the realm of science.

4. FALSE SCIENCE

'What!' some will say, 'do you then turn down the help science has to offer in the cause of justice? Has the Law got to remain purblind, uncertain, feeling its way among presumptions and probabilities? Must we, in order to preserve its traditional character, keep it always in the twilight of perpetual doubt?'

This point has not been overlooked in anything I have written. But it rests on a superstitious view of science. The true scientific spirit is to put science where it belongs and to make use of it only according to the amount of certainty it gives, and within the limits of that certainty. There is too much talk of science in this matter of narco-analysis. It is as if it sufficed to stick the label 'scientific' on a technique which, when all is said and done, is still untried and unproved, to impose it dogmatically upon both priests and faithful, not to mention its victims—in the temple of science.

1. Tahon, *op. cit.*

This is a new form of 'scientism', narrower and more dangerous than the scientific attitude of last century. It depends on the stupidity of the herd, the authoritarianism of its pontiffs, and on the acceptance of the right to use means which degrade man from his high estate. It claims to work under the aegis of *true* science, with its constant research, critical examination of hypotheses, careful affirmations, controls and all the rest, while in fact it is only *false* science, jumping prematurely to conclusions; a matter of passing fads, and of brutal and dictatorial assertions. It is now, if ever, when justice and equity are threatened, that one must refuse to be intimidated or taken in by such an imposture.

It is, anyway, wrong to submit to the general claims made by a contemporary science which is accepted uncritically by some, as an article of faith. It is *not* for science to regulate the universe and the affairs of man. Moreover, science itself does not have the right to self-rule : it exists for the service of man, and so, in its researches, as in the application of these researches, it has to be governed by superior moral ends which order it as they do all other forms of human activity. This is essential if civilization is to be protected from scientific barbarism. Man is not a subject for experimentation, no matter what possible good may accrue. The true reasons for using science are not to be gauged by its power, it effectiveness or even its certainty, but by its conformity with the moral standards and the spiritual dignity of man.

On the plane of law, where moral and spiritual good are at stake, this general principle becomes clear from the rule already stated, that a scientific method of investigation can be used in legal cases not only if it is really effective but primarily if it conforms to the spirit of justice. Further, even if its certainty and its safety were perfectly established, there is not necessarily any reason for applying such a method in a field where the factors involved are so complex that the use of a rigid and exact procedure can only result in an impoverishment of one's perspective, and a distortion of one's judgment. In every case the degree of exactitude sought for must fit the subject under consideration: to be too much or too little precise is to fail altogether in precision. If, for instance, it is true that there are such things as exact psychological tests, these may perhaps be usefully applied to vocational guidance. It would be most risky to use them to determine personal character and aptitudes, and ridiculous to try and assess spiritual aspirations or whether the subject has a religious vocation.

The same applies to the use of science in justice. If we assume that narco-analysis is an exact means of detecting deceit, that is still no reason for using it in trials. Matters are not so simple that everything said can be truly and easily assessed, even if the accused is proved to be a liar. It is a bad form of simplicity to treat by technical means problems which depend essentially on spiritual judgment. In fact, the more exact the technique, the more flagrant the mistakes will be. There are some lights which illumine: others merely dazzle.

What then of a method which is uncertain and flimsy, giving inconstant and inconsistent results, which is not particularly safe in use, and clearly not advisable in difficult cases involving serious problems? We have nothing against the therapeutic use of narco-analysis, apart from the doubts of some who use it. Even its more fervent advocates agree as to the variations in its effectiveness, according to the type of case and of the person receiving it. They speak of the great need of care both in preparing for it and in interpreting its results, and advise against its use by the inexperienced. They also warn the public against sensationalism and fantastic statements, and the belief that it is a quasi-magical system. On the contrary, it is already known to have only a narrow application and may soon find itself relegated to the museum of outworn medical fashions. This, on the clinical aspects of narco-analysis, where the patient is free and the aim is to heal. How much more should it apply to criminal cases, when it is used on a suspected person, and associated with punishment!

To speak too much of science in this matter is in any case to be skating on thin ice, for the best one can say about pentothal as already used in justice is that it was out of luck. Its first notable application resulted in a patent and monumental error. This error may, it is true, be due partly to the influence of the specific instructions received by the expert, which were to determine whether or not Cens was a malingerer. But this does not excuse pentothal so much as discredit it, since it suggests that it can be made to produce whatever results one wants. What is indeed certain is that it allowed those experts, ten months after their first attempt, the chance to contradict themselves directly, a fact which, if the whole matter were not so painful, might suggest an attitude of cheerful scepticism. For pentothal was responsible for the only diagnosis among the dozen or so made by experts on the miserable Cens, which contradicted every one made before and every one made after it was used. Who will believe that the simple use of pentothal gave the only accurate diagnosis, in straight contradiction to the conclusions drawn by careful observations and reached by classical methods, by all the other doctors? The first victim of this diagnosis is, of course, the accused man, whose sufferings were increased as a result. But pentothal itself suffers severely from its very first application, and it would take much to restore one's confidence in it.

5. THE PRINCIPLE OF INNER CONVICTION

All these claims of false science, these encroachments on the attributes of justice, arise from an inaccurate sense of the judicial act. Justice is not a technique. There is no exact method of determining intentions or of measuring responsibility and so doing away with the main work of the judge. This involves the assessment of contradictions, penetrating into and understanding spiritual matters by spiritual means.

Police methods may be scientific, and it is not to be denied that some of these, such as anthropometry and chemical and bacteriological analysis help one to pursue the search for and identification of delinquents. That is legitimate because one is looking for clues, not for intentions, to establish facts, not to draw conclusions and because after police investigation judicial trial must ensue.

The analysis of a drop of blood, the examination of a hair may allow the police to link a criminal act to its perpetrator. We are here face to face with a certain degree of scientific certainty, which can then be discussed. It does not invade and submerge the moral aspects of the debate. The judge may pay attention to this hair, but his assessment of the case as a whole will not depend entirely on it. The supposedly scientific operation which purports to detect lies or to measure responsibility is quite other, in that its conclusions are not factual but moral, and so tend to impose a ready-made conviction. Police science supplies a dossier of facts. Juridical science would foreclose the trial.

The greatest reservations must be made about the use of any form of mechanical lie-detector, such as those which have arisen out of the technical fertility of American imagination. The civilization of America has been described as passing without intermediate stages from the parrot to the gramophone stage. Its justice may be said to go from lynch-law to lie-detecting. In any case, the scientific value of such apparatus can lead to endless discussion. Some say that the margin of error is only 4%. Others opine that this low figure takes into account only the cases in which the mistakes are exposed, whereas the intrinsic quality of such errors is that they do not become apparent. It is also pointed out that skilled deceivers have learned to upset the workings of the machine, while frightened people, even if innocent, may register disturbances of much the same order as those of guilty people. Clearly, the judicial value of such apparatus is very dubious. They belong to police methods which no judge, at any rate in France (or in

Britain), would feel inclined to use even if he had the right to do so, because they infringe the moral code of true justice. To determine that a suspect is deceiving is a matter on which the judge must decide, taking into account the totality of the facts of the case. Nobody else taking part in the trial has the right to draw any such conclusion, especially if he does so only from a single source of information. If he does, the proceedings lack both judicial balance and scientific scepticism.

As to narcosis, its intrusion into the field of justice can become all the more dangerous from the scientific prestige it enjoys and by the fact that it is given by a doctor collaborating with the judge himself. It is hence given a sanction other than that of a police method, and so might bias the judge, giving him a sense of confidence it does not deserve, and so preventing him from the full use of his own inner intuitions. It could make justice a farce. The lie-detector may be a bad joke, but narco-analysis is supposed to belong to the realm of serious science, which is far more dangerous.

To reduce justice to a technique of psychic investigation is entirely contrary to the fundamental principles on which it rests to-day, that is, the inner, intuitive conviction of the judge. The notion of intuitive conviction is often interpreted in a bad light, and not without reason, for it has often been abused. Tribunals and juries have been constituted, whether for political or other purposes, of which the members, often inept, always badly prepared and instructed even to reach a reasonable conclusion, have given verdicts which were dubious, contradictory, and sometimes scandalously false, on the grounds that they represented their intuitive convictions. Such things have led to the association of the term with prejudice and hatred, and the bad odour of these partisan judgments has reflected against the idea of its use by the professional judge. People believe that the principle that the judge must act on his intimate convictions leads to arbitrary or erratic justice—to a happy-go-lucky régime.

Naturally, the advocates of scientific justice make great

play against it, and set themselves up as the crusaders of light and progress. All this is, however, due to misunderstanding. The principle of intuitive conviction can only be understood by comparison with the preceding rule, that of legal proof, which was in effect abolished in 1791. In this earlier system the legislature drew up a fixed schedule as to the values to be given to different forms of proof, so that the judgment was virtually calculated beforehand according to the stated weight of each piece of evidence brought forward. The judge had no need to weigh one against the other and decide which points are most important, and so to act on fine shades of discrimination. In this system, for instance, straight confession carried everything before it: it did not, as to-day, constitute only one of the items from which the judge has to form his convictions. No other proof was required, and sentence was pronounced accordingly. That such a system has some advantages must be admitted, since it furnishes a certain framework of judgment and to some extent counters the inconsistency and incompetence of a popular jury. This is especially true in Britain, yet it is well known that such a régime, despite the appearance of security it gives, by making the weighing of evidence impersonal, is no certain guarantee against a miscarriage of justice in particular cases.

This is because the need to obtain formal proof may urge the examining officer to try and obtain it at all costs (notably by forcing a confession), and hence leads to a deformation of the methods used for investigation (i.e. to tortures), and turns justice away from considering the inner values of that proof (even a confession may not be true). Moreover, the demand for proof may narrow the field of the judge's activities so much that he is no longer free to make his own appreciation of the facts, and force him to make a judgment which would not be really equitable. For if some legal proof appeared preponderant, it might oblige him to ignore others which should also be taken into account. If the fallacies of so rigid a system had not become apparent, it is doubtful whether the new philosophies of the Revolutionary period would alone have sufficed to decide on its abolition in favour of giving the last word to the supposedly infallible intuitions of the judge.

Compared with this form of strict juridical determinism, the principle of inner conviction is not, at any rate in the case of the professional judge, a giving way to haphazard methods. It does allow him freedom of appreciation, elasticity to compare and weigh evidence, and so to focus, to balance, to find shades of significance which, if one wishes to avoid mistakes, is essentially right for human beings making judgments on human affairs. He can then fit each element of proof into a whole, and so give it its true and therefore relative importance. The resulting judgment is thus made as solid as it can be, and it is backed by a moral conviction which should lead, not to the harshness of one made on proofs alone, but on an integration of many things.

The act of judging is thus defined: the judge is not an accountant charged with applying a general, universal, fixed schedule, but he is enabled to graduate his findings according to the circumstances of the act and the personality of the guilty party. Naturally, such a system may have its risks, but what complex human act of judgment is infallible? The risk can, moreover, be reduced by the use of extensive investigations as well as by the fact that in a Court of Law judgment depends on a group and not on a single person. Such a procedure admits the complexities of a case, and in human affairs the greatest source of error arises from over-simplification.

A system of justice claiming to be scientific must of necessity set the clock back and lead to another form of the false simplicity which we have outworn. That arising from the application of science would be in no way superior to that arising, as in the past, from over-abstract juridical principles. Superstitious faith in the absolute value of science here mingles with primitive evolutionary tendencies to predict the justice of the future: after the religious phase (trial by magic) comes the legalistic phase (predominant value given to confession of guilt), then the phase where intuitive conviction rules; and now we approach that of science, where the proof is to be determined by technique. It seems as if it were a dogma that science must automatically, and in every field, move in the direction of progress, yet in the field of justice, it could introduce factors which were nothing if not regressive.

Science used in this way would take the judge back to a rigid and mechanical system from which the principle of intuitive conviction has set him free. The price won by giving the judge freedom to work on this principle is that of a spiritualization of justice. From the art of simply recording facts, he is now allowed to examine these critically; from the application of scheduled verdicts and sentences, he can estimate the actual realities of the case; instead of acting automatically, he is made to act with careful and anxious consideration. It is surely essential that these things should be preserved and protected against techniques which claim to give peremptory proofs and ready-made conclusions.

The problem of the kind of collaboration which scientific techniques should have with matters of law is not easy. It really rests on the choice of those which can be admitted because they conform to this spirit of justice, respect the methods by which a case should be drawn up, the primacy of the judge and the principle of intuitive conviction.

Let me say again that this severe elimination of other methods will make justice lose nothing. On the contrary, these 'lights of science' by which we risk losing judicial traditions which have permanent moral value, are likely to fade out in a few years' time. The examining magistrate who used hypnosis not only transgressed the decencies of justice, but from the scientific viewpoint he was a fool. Without disrespect to the practitioners of narco-analysis— and Charcot was a great man—we must beware of falling into the same error.

Justice is not a scientific technique: it is a problem of conscience.

Chapter 6

THE CONFESSION DRUG

ACCUMULATION of argument has hidden the real problem, which now lies buried among fine points of distinction and euphemistic statements. The time has come to bring into the open the only real question, and to face it nakedly and frankly: pentothal as used in law is a drug which violates the mind of the individual and which obtains confessions by force.

Yes: confessions. On this point we must clear our minds of old pretences and equivocations. For the subtlest of subtle arguments is to argue that it is because pentothal has its weak points that we are prevented from finding a clear line beyond which the use of drugs and even of pentothal itself becomes an abuse. We are told we need not feel worried: narcosis does not provoke confessions of guilt, so we need have no fear of forcing confessions if we use pentothal for narcotizing the subject. This needs closer examination: *does* pentothal make people confess? And what kind of confession does it produce?

1. THE NATURE OF THE CONFESSION

Is pentothal an innocuous drug? If so, what are we to think either about it or the ideas of its advocates? Imported from America together with the opinions not only of its less competent partisans, but also with the backing of psychiatrists and criminologists, pentothal and similar drugs were first considered to be wonderful things, endowed with quasi-magical powers of exposing the real conscience: it *must* be used *because* it made people confess. It was not long before people changed their tune: pentothal does not *always* bring about confessions; it may give insignificant or untrue results. Anybody might have concluded that it is useless and even dangerous to use it for justice, and that it should be kept strictly for medical purposes. But not a bit of it! They do not give way but now say that it may safely be used since it does *not* result in confessions of guilt! This is a strange way of arguing from contradictory premises of the validity of the same conclusion! What, in short, is to be the final argument in favour of the use of narcosis in law : that one may expect everything from it, or else nothing ?

Some, of course, choose to propound both arguments at once; the same experts who justify narcosis as a means of reaching a diagnosis and aver that they would use it for no other purpose, declare that one need have no fear of it leading to an avowal of guilt. Yet at the same time they present narcosis as an infallible means of exposing lies, boasting that by its use they have definitely *proved* deception (and hence that it is much to be feared).[1] It is a kind of double game. In theory it is said that pentothal is a harmless aid to diagnosis, in practice it is admitted to be a fearful extortion drug. And when Dr. Heuyer says, '*The truth serum is humbug*,' should he mean by that that no expert would think of using it to make a suspect confess, then it is his own statement which becomes humbug. The expert investigation of which Cens was the victim had as its prime result that he was called a malingerer, because he 'confessed' that he was capable of pleading. How can anybody sincerely suggest that pentothal causes no confessions at the very moment when an expert bases his reports on a confession obtained by its use?

Let us now look at the facts. Is there anything in them which will enable us to know precisely whether or not pentothal produces true confessions of guilt? The first

1. Heuyer and Favreau, *op. cit.* (*Annales de méd. lég.*, March–April 1948, p. 102).

THE CONFESSION DRUG 103

thing which strikes one is the amount of uncertainty and disagreement.

We have already seen that practitioners discuss the degree of suggestibility and of lucidity of the patient. Some say he is very suggestible and highly receptive of ideas and persuasions put to him by the interrogator.[1] Others say his critical faculties and his memory are not diminished, that he remains entirely clear-minded, and that, without denying that his consciousness is affected by the drug because he is taken with *'an irresistible need to speak, to confess, to publicize his introspections.'*[2]

As to confessions, the uncertainty is even greater. In examining a number of cases, all of which, incidentally, are the outcome of attempts to detect malingering, one expert comes to the conclusion that narcosis *'has brought about no confessions among suspects who deny the accusations, nor any explanation of the facts which differs from that given in full consciousness while the system of mental defence is fully organized.'* At the same time as he affirms that *'defence reactions remain active'*, he recognizes *'a diminution of conscious and semi-conscious inhibitions, an increased demand for sympathy and a tendency to verbal expression which naturally tend to diminish the field of self-criticism.'*[3] When all is said and done, it seems difficult to believe that conscious control remains entirely unaffected.

Here, however, is another specialist, relying on equally extensive experience both of suspected people and of free subjects, who speaks of (1) certain cases where no admissions were obtained; (2) cases where, by uncontrolled answers, contradictions, half-admissions, alternations between 'Yes' and 'No', the subject gives himself away; and

1. Cossa, *op. cit.* (*Annales méd.-psych.*, Dec. 1945, p. 479), also Schneider, *op. cit.* (*Archives Suisses de neurologie et psychiatrie*, 1948, pp. 352 *et seq.*).

2. Cornil and Ollivier: *Problèmes de sélection et d'actualités médico-sociales*, pp. 145–146, and *Etudes de neuro-psychopathologie infantile*, p. 7.

3. Divry and Bobon, *op. cit.*, pp. 622–625.

(3) straight confessions from people who had already decided to keep silent at all costs, and who tried to evade even the most insidious questioning. The same writer says that, while himself under narcosis, he did not give exact details of what he wanted to hold back, but often gave himself away and said too much. He says that memory of very recent things is abolished under narcosis, and this is what enables one to trap the subject by clever and pressing questions, because he forgets what he has already said. The author also notes the sense of unease under narcosis, which is at times very strong, because the subject is aware of the attempt which is being made to break in on his mind, aggravated by the urge which he has to confess his guilt.[1]

Another worker reports a typical case of confession from a young soldier who claimed a pension for epilepsy, yet under narcosis, spontaneously owned that he had had fits since he was fifteen.[2] Underwood, in 1945, speaks of an American corporal court-martialled for murder and who, drugged with pentothal-sodium by an army psychiatrist, admitted his guilt.[3]

It amounts to this: that pentothal *may* bring about a confession, and another specialist[4] envisages its use one day, '*for the purpose of helping justice to obtain confessions from suspects*'.

Setting one opinion against another, it appears that the views of experts as to the value of narcosis are contradictory. Some say that the defence mechanisms of the subject remain active enough for a guilty person not to confess and to pass himself off as innocent,[5] while others, who propose

1. Schneider, *loc. cit.*, pp. 352 *et seq.*
2. Cossa, *op. cit.*, p. 456.
3. Divry and Bobon, *loc. cit.*, pp. 610–611. In general, these two experts, who try and minimize the danger of pentothal as a confessional drug, nevertheless report many examples of the use of drugs as a means of forcing admissions.
4. Trillot, *op. cit.* (*Acta med. leg. et soc.*, p. 653).
5. This is the opinion of Divry and Bobon and also of Schneider—*op. cit.*

to use pentothal to justify innocence seem, on the contrary, to believe that only the innocent can maintain silence.[1]

On these various indications it seems difficult to accept the reassuring statement that pentothal will *never* force a confession of guilt. The contrary, in fact, is proved. And if it is true that the lack of unanimity among practitioners is due to the diversity of results in individual cases, this only goes to prove that we are in the presence of a drug of which we do not yet really know the qualities. These qualities are sometimes harmless, sometimes the reverse, and consequently we cannot accept that it be used as a drug to force unwilling confessions.

What exactly is the meaning of the word 'confession' in this context? If one means by it true statements about material facts, then pentothal may sometimes make a person confess, at other times not. But there are also indirect confessions, and pentothal can bring these about by producing revealing signs and actions which signify and are equivalent to confession.

We have already spoken of the half-admissions and the contradictions which trip the subject up and make him give himself away. There are other cases where, despite apparent control and persistent denials, the subject under the influence of a barbiturate changes the tone of his statements and only denies mildly what hitherto he denied with vehemence. Returning to the two reports made by Professor Delay to the Medico-legal Society, it appears that neither subject admitted responsibility for the acts of which he was accused. They continued to deny; but one said, '*There are some things one cannot tell*,' the other, '*I remember when I want to, but not when I do not*': an obvious change of attitude from straight denial to evasive replies which might easily be looked upon as confession. In how many cases might one not find, under narcosis, this weakening of the strength of the denials?

1. Cornil and Ollivier: *Problèmes de sélection et d'actualités méd.-sociales*, pp. 150–151.

How, moreover, can anybody affirm that narcosis never gives admissions of guilt, yet that it is useful in the systematic unmasking of deceit? Here indeed is indirect confession, and a feature more important than direct admissions, for it is a general matter and applies not only to a specific act but to the whole behaviour of the subject. How does one unmask a deceiver otherwise than by forcing him to admit himself a liar? Under the euphemism of 'showing up deceit' lies concealed the fact that one is actually seeking out lies, against the wishes of the subject, even without his being aware that this is being done.

It seems as if during the pentothal test among malingerers, certain conscious psychic contents, hitherto strongly concealed, remain concealed, but the subject, unknown to himself and to his wish to dissemble, gives himself away, and sometimes gives information of facts he hid while in full consciousness.[1]

Can this be called using pentothal for anything else than for obtaining confessions, whether directly or indirectly?

Let us not forget too that the alleged harmlessness of pentothal by no means guarantees anything as to the future. We know that pentothal is only a beginning and that there are already means of making its effects more drastic if one chooses. The intrinsic properties of the drug are, anyway, less important than the motives which govern its use. The one who is determined to obtain a confession or to show up a lie knows very well what drug to add if pentothal alone is not effective. The way to Avernus is open, and science—if one may speak of science in this connection, where as soon as a technique claims to wear the label 'scientific' it is thought that it may be used for any purpose —is always adding to the arsenal of drugs which can be employed for assault. There is already a perfected technique of narcosis. Here is what Professor Delay writes as a warning against abuses:

Gradual narcosis with amytal, followed by a sudden

1. Delay, *op. cit.*, p. 66.

awakening by the use of benzedrine, makes the verbal objectivization of psychic contents most urgent and they come with an explosive force hitherto unknown.'[1]

One guesses the horrible reality under the specialist's jargon.

It is doubtless the sense that they are starting on a sinister road, the end of which cannot be foreseen, which makes some of the more enlightened and scrupulous advocates of pentothal take up a hesitant and cautious attitude. On the one hand they say, that '*it would be regrettable if modern methods of investigation were to be prohibited*', while on the other they declare that '*pentothal must not become the truth serum*', that it must not be used to extort confessions. The protest is useless, for a resolution is no prohibition, and only shows the anxiety which every true scientist must feel at the prospect of one day losing control of his inventions, or seeing techniques originally intended for man's good, used instead for his undoing. The advocates of pentothal are indeed playing the rôle of sorcerer's apprentices.

2. UNTRUE CONFESSIONS

Still the advocates of narcosis persist. Their ultimate argument puts the final touch to our astonishment. This is when they insist—with truth—on the uncertainties of narcosis and that, despite the current view based on the unfortunate phrase, 'truth serum', pentothal has no magic powers. They also say, with equal truth, that its effect is to produce a mass of contradictory and uncertain statements which requires expert sorting out and criticism. Despite all this, they claim that there is nothing to fear from it! For how can anybody believe that any expert should have thought of using it to obtain confessions, or that it might be used as a method of police enquiry? In short, say this group, pentothal is harmless *because* it misleads!

1. Delay: *Le pentothal ne doit pas devenir le sérum de vérité* (*Figaro*, 12 Nov. 1948).

This is certainly different from saying that narcosis forces confession and that this confession is true. The second part of this proposition has never been seriously believed except perhaps by the first American pioneers to use scopolamine and pentothal, and later by a public which took literally and blindly to the expression, 'truth serum'. We may remember the caution against taking this phrase seriously and without coupling with it the irony and scepticism implied by the Latin proverb, *in vino veritas*. We saw how there was reason to fear that the 'truth' obtained by pentothal might be befuddled, and that the confessions it gave might be false: which is yet a further reason for keeping it away from judicial procedures.[1]

Here, however, we have a curious *volte face*, in which an attempt is made to discredit the opponents of pentothal by trying to make them out to be over-credulous. It is said that those who are afraid of seeing pentothal used in law are sufficiently naïve to believe in the truth serum, to take at face value the statements of journalists that true confessions can be obtained. Hence, they are supposed to believe that it is able to strip the mind to a state of primitive nakedness. This is nonsense on the part of the fearful, since we have to do with a highly scientific method, the very complexity of which is a safeguard against inexpert use.

> Only the professional psychoanalyst is fit to interpret the things said during wakening, to catch their exact meaning, which is often obscure and symbolic. . . . It is a dangerous operation, full of possible mistakes. It is naïve to fear its use by the police.[3]

Have we not already been told that the truth serum is humbug, a thing we know only too well since it was by one of its mistakes that the lot of a poor wretch was made much worse? This shows well enough that the need for 'interpretation of symbols' is not a sufficient safeguard. Policemen

---

1. Jean Rolin: *Le pentothal, drogue de l'aveu* (*Etudes*, Oct. 1948).
2. Mellor: *La Torture*, p. 283.

are not usually interested in symbolic meanings, and their use of 'third degree' methods are designed simply to bring about straight, unsymbolic confessions. It is this very tendency which has made justices anxious about the matter, and which is a peremptory reason for prohibiting the use of such methods. Can 'third degree' and other tortures be condemned because of the errors which arise from them, while on the other hand condoning the use of pentothal because it too results in inaccuracy? If the confessional drug is full of possible mistakes, that is no reason for reassurance in its use. On the contrary, it is doubly to be dreaded since it not only violates one's conscience but makes one confess to what one has not done. Truth serum? Surely not: lie serum, rather!

It scarcely seems necessary to enlarge again on the numerous risks of distortion which arise from a procedure which alters the personality of the subject by affecting his consciousness, and which may mislead even experienced practitioners, let alone others, and so may cause flagrant miscarriages of justice. All users of the drug agree on the alteration of consciousness which it produces, though all do not agree on the degree to which this occurs. Even those who affirm that the lucidity of many cases is increased and that they are hypermnesic and keep all their powers of self-criticism,[1] do not deny the 'toxic grip'. Can one admit that every act and word resulting from alcoholic intoxication shows a psychological basis of fact? What if, as some writers say, one admits that extreme suggestibility of the hypnogogic state creates a situation in which the least emphatic question may suggest the theme of the answer? If even expert practitioners have to use such care, it is easy to see what might happen in unscrupulous hands: one might be able to make anybody admit to anything, at least in words.

Even without pressure or suggestions, false confessions

1. Cornil and Ollivier: *Problèmes de sélection et d'actualités médico-sociales*, pp. 144, 146–147.

may occur. One knows the delirium of self-accusation sometimes found in drunkenness, when the subject accuses himself, in great detail, of misdeeds he has not committed, while others boast of quite fictitious exploits. There is the same lack of affective inhibitions, the need to 'spill the beans', to talk without reserve which is typical also of barbiturate narcosis, and where false confessions are just as likely. Any psychopathic case, brooding over a guilt-complex, is likely to behave like this, for in the realm of the unconscious mind, which is liberated from control by pentothal, the frontier between factual and imagined realities is uncertain. When the unconscious comes to the surface, the imaginary and the real may, in the eyes of a person under narcosis, become tinged with the same colours.[1]

Even in normal people the risk of false confessions is not entirely excluded. Any repressed desire or wish may come to the surface as if it had been satisfied. All the monsters which sleep in the depths of the consciousness of honest men, and primarily those of guilt for things he has never wished or dared to commit, morbid fantasies of pleasures or of pain, lost occasions for sin—all these may come out as compensatory hallucinations under pentothal. Each one may say that he has actually done what he may only have wished to do, and even a saint could not be sure that images of rejected temptations might not assail him as if they were the ghosts of real sins. Thus there is no innocence under pentothal which does not become suspect. This applies especially to the worst of these unconscious monsters, because they cause most anxiety and so are those most carefully concealed and guarded.

On the other hand, there is the case of the shameless rogue, hardened to crimes for which he does not feel any guilt, and further protected by the psychological simplicity of the primitive brute. He also has a strong nervous resistance to the effects of drugging, and is altogether

[1]. Delay, *loc. cit.* (*Figaro*, 12 Nov. 1948), and *Les aveux artificiels* (*Figaro*, 11 Feb. 1949).

invulnerable in matters of conscience. Pentothal will dislodge him neither from malingering nor lying, and he will emerge from narcosis with a certificate of innocence and a report of a character as white as snow. Pentothal will make the innocent confess to what they have not actually done, but will not make the guilty admit their crime. This is the ridiculous story of the American mechanical lie-detector : the tough are not caught out by it, the innocent are.

So from a purely medical standpoint, confessions obtained by drugging are valueless and do not give grounds for determining responsibility. One may even go further and suggest that there is an *a priori* doubt attached to any confession made under narcosis, unless this is checked and confirmed in waking consciousness. Ignorance of this rule was the chief source of error in the expert's reports on Cens, and was due to a direct transposition from what the mind showed under narcosis to what it showed under normal conditions: it was assumed that if a subject could speak under pentothal he could also speak before the examining magistrate, and the reasons he gave for his silence were held as additional proof of this. In truth, all these data from an altered personality should have been doubted. If care had been taken to verify the diagnosis when he was in his normal state, as was done later by other experts, it would have been seen that none of the conclusions drawn were justified. By causing psychic collapse, the drug immediately casts doubts on the results which it is going to give.

3. THE PREJUDICE IN FAVOUR OF CONFESSION: THE USE OF TORTURE

Since pentothal can lead to errors in the psychological sphere, to what others can it not lead in the forensic? In the use of such a drug, a mistake in principle, which then becomes the mother of all subsequent mistakes, stands out as first to be condemned: that is, the search at all costs for an admission of guilt. A form of justice starting on this road is liable to find itself on any number of false tracks and misconceptions, while the experts who consider it their rôle to outwit deception and who believe themselves to be up-to-date are in reality pushing justice backward to the time when confession was taken as paramount, and as sufficient proof of guilt.

We know what an abuse torture is when used in search of a confession. But it is used for other reasons too. It shows in the torturer himself a liking for making others suffer, and arises from primitive sadism which no degree of civilization has yet been able to uproot entirely from the heart of man, and which is apt to rear its ugly head again in times of anarchy. Yet torture is not only an anarchical regression towards the sadism of the barbarian. For a long time it was an institution of the judicial system, and even Christianity did not prevail against it. Centuries passed between the protests of St. Augustine and those of Voltaire and its official abolition. During all that time, serious and honest men, judges, magistrates and inquisitors, about whom the explanation of simple sadism is inadequate, presided without a shudder at some of the greatest scenes of horror in all history, confident in the dignity of their function and with a sense of duty done. In the undoubtedly civilized country of ancient France, and in the carefully elaborated framework of judicial institutions, this was certainly a monstrous anomaly.

A single explanation is enough to cover the fact of judicial torture, so different at any rate in its conscious motives from plain sadism, and that is, the legal tyranny of proof by confession. Torture became an institution owing to the degree in which such confession was held to be the ultimate proof of guilt.

It would not be true to say that the jurists of olden times were unaware of the danger that injustice might arise from the use of torture. Their objections to it—and they are

THE CONFESSION DRUG

more numerous than one might suppose—arose not only from pity and human feeling, but they agreed that mistakes were caused by untrue admissions made under torture. '*A thousand and a thousand have loaded themselves with false confessions*,' wrote Montaigne. Moreover, it is evident that the ability to stand up to torture is not proportional to one's innocence and, according to a phrase of La Bruyère, it is '*an invention which is certain to condemn an innocent person whose constitution is weak, but to save a guilty one who is born tough.*' So that even the old system of jurisprudence made reservations in its insistence on the value of confession. Torture was only to be applied after certain prior indications were found, confession alone was not held to be an absolute proof and involved capital punishment only if the evidence of a good witness supported it. And, in any case, the confession could be retracted and only carried full weight if freely confirmed. In short, one may put it that there was a certain degree of civilization even about torture, a general procedure aiming, if not at humanizing such barbarous methods, at any rate at doing away with the worst judicial errors it might cause.

The basic flaw nevertheless remains in the motives behind its use, the insistence on obtaining a confession. Whatever variations there may be in technique it is this which really explains judicial torture. One may call it *the spirit of torture*, and it is established that the use of torture in law only vanished from French institutions (by a decree of Louis XVI in 1780), when forensic ideas, gradually evolving over centuries, and reaching a climax when the system of legal proof disappeared, became ready to place confessions among other items of evidence in criminal cases. It thus gave admissions of guilt a relative, no longer an absolute value, and allowed the judge a measure of discretion he had not got under the tyranny of the older system. Conversely, one still sees that in places where the main concern is to obtain a confession, the spirit and the practice of torture remain. No other explanation need be sought to explain the brutalities and abuses which are the shame of any police force. Apart from the pleasure and morbid satisfaction felt by some in holding a man at their mercy, one must not attribute to a general sadistic spirit the use of police methods which the best of them vigorously repudiate. The real reason is—as still taught in certain police manuals[1]—that police interrogation aims primarily at being effective—and to be effective means to obtain a confession. This is taken as a justification for improper procedures, but in fact it side-tracks the policeman from his proper function, which is not to pounce on his suspect as a prey to be questioned, but to establish facts and collect evidence before they disappear. Note also that few policemen have the legal or psychological wisdom which teaches them to be cautious about confessions, and not to take them as categorical proofs. It is clear that such people may find themselves driven to pursue a confession and, if the person under interrogation resists, they may become torturers from exasperation. So long as the function of the police is not clearly defined as being not that of extractors of confessions, but finders of facts, it remains useless to decry 'third degree' methods and interrogations lasting forty-eight hours. Judicial torture can only be abolished when the spirit of torture is also abolished.

These considerations clarify both the comparison of pentothal to torture and the danger to justice which goes with the use of that drug. It may be too hasty, but it is not altogether wrong, to say that legalistic narcosis is a new form of torture. It is not what is commonly called torture since the technique of its use is not an atrocious and refined way of inflicting suffering, but on the contrary, produces a state of euphoria. Neither can one say that, on the subjective plane, narcosis is a form of sadism, nor that its advocates are low-grade inquisitors. Yet the use of narcosis in the obstinate pursuit of confession is a revival of the forensic

1. See Lambert (*op. cit*), from whom Maître Mellor quotes (in *La Torture*, pp. 273 *et seq*.) the strange theory of *legitimate tortures*.

attitude behind the use of torture. In the case of the Belgian traitor, pitilessly pursued with a syringe and mercilessly drugged with various products; in the Cens case, where pentothal upset a diagnosis already certain; in the claim that the *prime* goal of mental *expertise* is to show up liars, we have clear indications of a regression to the time when torture was acceptable in law. If there is now no suffering to the patient, no sadism in the one who inflicts it, there is nevertheless the spirit of torture in the legal mind which supports it. Modern and honourable judges and experts to-day are no more monsters than were their predecessors. Like them, they fulfil their function with the dignity of their profession. Yet, of old, these same honourable judges ordered that horrors be performed; and the honourable experts to-day are by way of practising other horrors, not to be compared with the older cruelties, but similar in their motivation. Even the skill at euphemism is there. The older magistrates decently disguised what they did by calling it 'questioning'; equally serious experts to-day dub it 'diagnosis'.

The danger of pentothal in reintroducing the relentless pursuit of confession is even greater than that of sadistic torture and needs even clearer condemnation. Sadistic torture is a horrible thing which naturally repels any decent person: the very facts, when known, arouse detestation, and when it is brought out from secret dungeons and dark cellars into the light of day, all its hideousness becomes apparent. But pentothal works indirectly to the same ends, supported by subtle and insidious arguments, and by the ignorance of the public. It is trying to establish itself as a recognized and regularly used procedure, but under the mantle of judicial dignity and with the prestige of science, it may easily put the clock of justice back towards the worst forms of extortion, and that all the more easily because it evokes neither pity on account of suffering nor disgust with the torturer who works insidiously and accomplishes by gentle means what he would not dare to do by brutality.

It is right to condemn obvious forms of torture. It would be fatal if we made the mistake of letting them be reintroduced in disguised and seemingly gentlemanly forms.

4. A FORENSIC CRITICISM OF CONFESSION

We have therefore to go to the very root of the evil, that of the overwhelming value of the confession of guilt, which originally inspired the use of torture, and which medical experts are trying to revive to-day. In the light of forensic criticism of the value of confession it is safe to say that the pretensions of pentothal must finally collapse.

The factual inaccuracy of admissions of guilt are very frequent. Without speaking of the sincere but erroneous confession made by a person whose memory of the reasons and circumstances of his actions is bad, there are, as we have seen, many forms of entirely false avowal made by people who plead guilty to things they have never done. For this there are many reasons. A suspect may make a false admission under duress, threats, torture; or under the influence of sentiments such as the hope of leniency, or of affection for another person from whom he wishes to remove suspicion; from the desire to show off; from despair. There are also pathological factors, suggestibility and self-guilt. We have also indirect, tacit false confessions, a guilty appearance, evasive glances, difficult speech, emotionalism, lying, muteness, all of which need careful assessment since they may occur in a person who is nothing more than innocently nervous.

In the light of this it must be realized that confession alone counts for nothing. It has to be taken together with other proofs, evidence, statements of witnesses, to be seen as part of a whole. We have already shown that pentothal may make the work of criticizing these doubly difficult, first by multiplying the chances of false admissions from emotional or suggestible people, and also by giving the experts' conclusions as to intention to deceive an over-dominant place.

Some legal experts have become so suspicious as to confessions that they wish to allow it no value in proof and want to do away with any attempt to reach it when considering a case.[1] This would, of course, be the best means of doing away with the exorbitant importance allowed in the proceedings to the results of interrogation, and to cut short the usurpations and abuses which arise from it. The idea of abolishing the interrogation is a wide judicial problem which does not belong here. But there is a risk that in our field such an extreme measure might lead to new dangers. For if, in theory, no account is to be taken of a confession of guilt, this might only serve as a pretext to reintroduce, by roundabout ways, methods of seeking a confession which would not be recognized as such. Under cover of the idea that confession is of no importance, it would be possible to give force to indications which would seem to hint at an indirect admission of guilt.

The legal problem about confession is not actually solved by refusing altogether to consider it as evidence, for this might lead to a compensatory bias in the case. It is safer to give it its just and proper place in the proceedings. If it was allowed its right value, neither more nor less, among the pleadings as a whole, it would do away with the obstinacy of policeman or doctor to force open the victim's consciousness. Pentothal would lose at once its importance and its pretensions, for if confession is neither essential nor sufficient by itself, neither will be the drug which is said to bring it about.

The forensic value of confession rests not only on its factual exactness but also on the conditions and the state of mind in which it was made. Even if it is entirely accurate it may have no value in law. This would be the case if pentothal were used. Only a confession voluntarily and deliberately made, knowing what it comports, by a person in full possession of his faculties can really carry the weight of

---

1. Maître Garçon: Report to the *Société des Prisons*, 1928.

proof. The more spontaneously it is made, the better, both because confession under torture is not likely to be accurate and also because it obscures the mental state and the motives behind the acts it admits. It is impossible to know whether the one who confesses under constraint is doing so only from fear, or whether he has any sense of guilt and responsibility for his crime, from dread of the judge, or in a spirit of repentance. It has no value if it does not show the state of the conscience of the accused, and stands as an integral aspect of his personality. Only so does it help to measure the degree of responsibility for the act.

To make such a measurement it is necessary to know both the psychological motives which led to an admission (e.g. release of nervous tension, the need to excuse oneself, inability to lie convincingly, exhibitionism, despair), the form in which it was expressed (vague; detailed; by a simple gesture; spontaneous; or in answer to leading questions; and so on); also the emotions shown when it was being made, and which give it moral significance (i.e. whether done blindly or with consciousness of guilt, cynicism or shame). Let us note in passing that if the police were told to report no confessions without at the same time stating the influences and circumstances under which the suspected person made them, this might well prevent them from using improper forms of interrogation, as well as strengthening the critical demands of the judges.

The need, already emphasized, to treat confession as a single act of a whole personality implies the option to withdraw it at any time before the conclusion of the trial. This withdrawal must, of course, be considered in the same light as the confession itself and its value looked upon as exactly its opposite—i.e. if the confession was made under duress or unwittingly, its retraction should be allowed to carry full weight in favour of the accused, whereas it becomes all the more important against him if the admission of guilt was freely made.

If this principle is admitted, narcosis clearly stands condemned, since the only confessions obtained under it take place in a state of disturbed consciousness and without the control of the self. In such a case, retraction of the confession should be allowed to stand in his favour.

Add to this that from a strictly judicial standpoint the only valid confession is that made before a judge or magistrate. It follows that one made to a medical man is legally void, just as it is if it were made to the police during interrogation. This gives the final touch to the reasons for not allowing pentothal, by altering the personality of the subject, to bring to light the contents of his mind in any way which may suggest, whether directly or indirectly, that he had pleaded guilty to his crime.

And, once more, no roundabout justification should be allowed for its use on the grounds that, if confession under pentothal is invalid, it does not matter if it is obtained. For this would imply that the judge's intuitions were absolutely, and entirely safe from being influenced by any legally dubious suggestion. It has taken many public scandals before judges finally realized the unworthy methods used by certain policemen in order to obtain confessions, and, further, to cast doubt on their credibility—and that despite the fact that they are technically worthless. It may take many more before it is finally decided that the law must be strictly respected, and policemen threatened with penalties should they use means of questioning which they have simply usurped. The same may have to happen with pentothal, should it become a feature of judicial procedure, before it can be finally dethroned from exerting any influence on the mind of the judge.

5. THE MORAL SIGNIFICANCE OF CONFESSION

All this legal criticism ultimately rest on principles of morality. For if justice demands that the only revelations which should carry weight are those freely made by a person in his normal state, this means that certain basic moral considerations are involved, which alone can make a confession valid.

Confession has no human value unless it is made by a person acting freely while in full possession of his faculties. It must be so, not only to give the facts accurately, but also to place the act correctly in regard to the personality of the suspect: was the crime committed with deliberate intent or in a state of passion, from passing emotion or ingrained habit, callously or with immediate regrets? In every real confession there is implied a possibility of classifying the action in the hierarchy of thoughts and wishes, and to see how deeply rooted were the motives in the mind of the subject—in short, to understand what exactly is his moral responsibility. It is obvious that narcosis has no respect for the conditions of such determination which make such a confession useful, since, by general admission, it is apparent that it acts by removing self-control and confusing the proper order of the elements making up the subject's consciousness. In this way a confession becomes nothing more than a form of mental purging.

So confession must be free if it is to have any moral and regenerative force. But if the only purpose of obtaining one is in order to deal with the material facts, to chase the suspect until he collapses and so can be destroyed like a wild beast, simply because of the outer appearances of his deed, then, no doubt, any expedient, including the use of pentothal, is valuable. But civilized society does not see things in this light, and when a judge says to a suspect, 'Confess or we shall take account of your refusal', this is surely more than a trick of bargaining so as to obtain more hold on the victim. When it is said that confession lightens the burden of a crime, this does not apply only to the physical relief of the man tired out with defending himself, since this would only deal with the outermost aspects of the matter.

Every form of confession—and this can be as validly said

of the sacramental form as of a declaration of love—is an act of self-abandonment in which are tacitly or openly expressed the most deeply moving things which a free person can say to another: '*I put myself in your hands, I give you power over myself*'. The confession made by a person accused of a crime and hence in an uncomfortable position, can never have the degree of freedom and spontaneity of the avowal either of a penitent or a lover, but it nevertheless retains some element of the same self-surrender and hence of a kind of reconciliation between himself and his judge. Conversely, the judge can no longer treat a suspect who has confessed exactly as he did before, because the two are no longer in opposite camps. The judge should respond to this self-abandonment as to a request for help: here is no longer a wild beast to be destroyed but a man he has taken under his care. In so far as this reconciliation shows either explicitly or unconsciously that the accused recognizes that he has transgressed moral values, it represents a step forward in the expiation and the moral reinstatement which any justice worthy of the name must—even without delving into psychic depths—be ready to consider, to allow, and in fact to aim at.

Unless the subject is acting as a free agent, a confession leads to nothing more than a lowering of man's estate, if he gives way from fear, constraint or torture. Confession under pentothal is a surrender to force or to trickery, a surrender even of the freedom whether to surrender or not: so it is a double degradation. The spiritual drama of co-operation between minds, which is the deep meaning of truly humane justice, is reduced by it to nothing more than a bestial fight in which all means may be used provided they result in a kill.

Chapter 7

THE SANCTITY OF SECRECY

THE foregoing criticism of the principles behind confession now takes us to the spiritual basis of my opposition to the use of pentothal.

1. THE RIGHT TO KEEP SILENT

There is a fundamental principle in criminal procedure which stands behind both the use of confessions and the search for confession. This is the right of the accused to refuse to answer questions. This right was only secured gradually, after the abolition of torture, and its revocation would carry justice into the worst of aberrations.

The right to silence has not always been granted. The old oath administered to a suspect used to put on him a moral compulsion—i.e. an indirect form of constraint—not only not to tell lies but also to speak the truth; if he did not do so, he would be breaking his oath and thereby incurring extra sanctions. The regulations issued in France in 1670 prescribed penalties against one 'mute of malice', and allowed judges to hold as proved accusations on which he refused to speak.[1] Similarly, failure to appear in court, or flight, was—as it tends to be to-day—taken as a sure sign of guilt.

This was so despite the principle that nobody could be forced to accuse himself—and hence to answer questions—

---

1. *Cf.* the oath administered to-day in British Courts, where the witness makes the impossible promise to speak 'The whole truth'. A prisoner on trial who elects to go into the witness-box is thereby bound to accuse himself, whereas if he does not give evidence, some measure of suspicion is cast on him by his refusal.—*Tr*.

THE SANCTITY OF SECRECY

already contained in Roman Law in the maxim: *nec enim aequum est dolum suum quemquam revelare*. English Common Law has accepted this for a long time. It was only in the nineteenth century that it was readopted in Continental European Law, and modern Canon Law confirms this implicitly in Article 1743: the parties are expected to answer the judge's questions and to tell the truth *unless it concerns a crime any of them may have committed*. French procedure adopted this in a law of 8 December 1897 and made it obligatory for the magistrate to warn the accused of his right to keep silent. If other codes of law do not formally emphasize the need for this caution, they all accept implicitly or in practice the principle of freedom to speak or keep silent.

The justification of such freedom is the very one which condemns the use of torture. For an accused person may be forced under constraint to admit to any crime, and hence the value of what he says is diminished. It is easier for a judge to imply the truth behind his silence from other indications and evidence than it is to avoid mistakes by listening to false or fantastic declarations.

In law, the right to keep silent is a logical corollary to the general principle of presumed innocence. It is for the prosecution to prove its charges, and the accused cannot be made to give proof of his innocence for the plain reason that he would very often not be able to do so. Innocence is a negative state and, like other negatives, cannot be positively proved except sometimes indirectly by an alibi. An accused person cannot logically be forced to speak when it may be that he has nothing to hide, and so nothing to speak about.

On the moral plane it seems more difficult to justify the right to silence, for it may be held that the accused ought to tell the truth, and that justice has every right to try and obtain it. Casuists have of course considered this argument, yet even they have agreed that confession must be left entirely free, though it would be difficult to find complete rational justification for this opinion: rather is it like the moral intuitions of the Church expressed by general agreement among theologians and which henceforth becomes a rule for interpretation. It must of course not be held to legitimize lying: it is a simple acknowledgement of a secret conflict which cannot be resolved by geometric propositions. The casuists leave the suspect free in his choice between silence and confessing the truth. While they acknowledge as a perfect solution that a guilty person should spontaneously offer himself up to whatever punishment he deserves, they consider that such heroism is beyond what may be expected of human beings and that it would be inhuman to demand that a man should set to work to condemn himself. In this way allowance is made for the frailty of man.

Needless to add, the right to keep silent does not confer immunity on the accused: he is using a right which is not an excuse nor a means of escaping justice. The refusal of a suspect to speak does not stop the prosecution from looking for evidence; on the contrary, since it may mean that he is hiding something, it becomes suspicious and consequently stimulates the search for whatever his silence may be covering. It will not, however, do to take silence as proof because, like confession, it may have as many implications as there are states of mind to motivate it. It is useful to know here too whether it is due to cynicism, callousness, charity to another, embarrassment or shame. Some silences may arise from considered attitudes (such as those we shall discuss, in front of judicial improprieties) and these may be more noble than confessions due to fear, boasting or calculation. This is all the more reason for respecting, while at the same time taking into consideration, the absolute right of the accused not to speak but to retire into the sanctuary of his innermost conscience. Can a further step be justified? If the accused has the right not to speak, it may be argued that he has the positive right to lie. For, it may be said, his right in the matter of confession is held to be so complete that he can refuse to admit his guilt not only by the default of silence, but by the positive act of lying and making false statements. The problem is not so simple as it looks; nevertheless its solution is the same.

On the moral plane, it would be saying too much, and saying the wrong thing, to speak of a *right* to tell lies. It is obvious that pure lying can be no more ethical in a court of justice than it is elsewhere, and so it is not a legitimate weapon of defence. Saint Thomas declares unequivocally that a suspect sins when he lies to the judge. At the same time it is certain that if the basic thesis is accepted in practice that no man should be compelled to condemn himself, it cannot be restricted simply to the right to keep silent since in some cases this might be a sure way of admitting himself guilty. He must also be allowed the right to deny. False denial—or active lying—is for all practical purposes inseparable from silence or passive lying.

Legally, moreover, its justification is the same. The freedom to keep silent and the freedom to lie are not so much real *rights*, resting on conscience and logically defensible, they are really human *powers* and not to be classed with the unacceptable forms of abuse which might arise were they to be disallowed. To say that a suspect can lie is not the same as to say he is doing right by lying, and that he is not transgressing moral principles. It is, however, to admit that he has a certain power of self-defence against violation of his consciousness and against extortion, that others have no right to know what he has in his mind except what can be discovered by normal means which neither infringe his liberty of choice nor alienate his normal personality. The thing which stands untouched against this is the right of the judge to circumvent and to see through lies. If he has the right to convict a person of lying, he has, however, no right to abolish his power to do so. He may point out the evidence implicit in his silence, his emotional manifestations, his half-admissions, his self-contradictions, but he has no right to obliterate at its source the freedom of choice of which the telling of a lie is simply a practical application—morally pernicious no doubt, but juridically sacrosanct.

Yet another step, and we return once more to the aggravating yet dominant question of malingering. If a suspect has the right to keep silent or to lie, must he also be allowed the particular kind of lie which consists in feigning mental sickness in order to escape questioning, and so to try and diminish the degree of responsibility to be attributed to him? Here, the points of view of morality and of law are complicated by that of medicine.

We know that the problem is rarely simple, and that malingering is often a semi-diseased condition, not a straightforward and simple attempt to deceive. Because its root lies in the pathological sphere, it comes outside the purely forensic field of the power to lie, and requires a medical assessment of the respective factors, voluntary lying and involuntary or pathological lying, of which it consists.

Nevertheless, in so far as there is voluntary and deliberate lying by any individual, malingering is merely making use of the power to lie which, as we have seen, cannot properly be proscribed. One cannot differentiate between lying and malingering by calling the latter an act of legal contempt, since lies are also attempts to outwit the judge. Malingering is merely a lie by action. Like verbal lying, malingering must also be held to be within the framework of what is allowable; and if this is so before the judge, it is equally so before the doctor who acts under the judge's instructions. Hence, when faced by deliberate or supposedly deliberate malingering, and all the more so if there is good cause to think and not only to suspect that it may be deliberate, there is greater reason for the expert to abstain from using means which destroy the freewill of the individual by paralysing his very ability to defend himself by deceit. For, on general principles he has no more authority than the judge to compel the subject to speak, or, by altering his personality, to prevent him from using that conscious control which enables him to malinger just as it enables him to keep silent.

Naturally, to allow a man to lie does not mean that one has to be taken in by him, and both expert and judge have the right to interpret any indications presented to them. Just as a judge may confound a liar by showing up his inconsistencies, so may a doctor prove by his analysis, or by his examination of nervous reflexes and the like, that the accused is feigning an illness he has not got. By so doing he is finding actual evidence, he is not violating the *intentions* of the patient. This is a distinction of primary importance to which we shall have to return. Its value is that it clarifies a serious confusion. For it is asserted that the unmasking of deception by pentothal is in the same category as that done by clinical examination: reflex actions being uncontrollable by the patient, to stimulate a reflex is to violate the freewill of the subject: hence, if examination of nervous reflexes is allowable, so is narcosis.[1] One might equally argue that a judge is just as much violating the freewill of the accused by showing up his contradictions and lies as by submitting him to torture, and hence that torture is as permissible as is the dialectic skill of the prosecution. Reflexes are like questions: objective manifestations which can be interpreted. If the reflexes are normal one can conclude to the insincerity of a malingerer just as one can if he lies badly. One has, in either case, shown up the lie; but one has not prevented him from lying.

This gives a clear line of demarcation between diagnosis and extortion—a thing which many experts have so far failed to see. Just like judicial interpretation, medical diagnosis should be carried out by interpretation of signs, not by direct attack against the freewill of the individual. It is no longer a diagnosis or a judicial examination when means are used which go beyond the detection of signs but which bring pressure to bear on the subjective power to manifest these signs or not. In conclusion: pentothal is *ipso facto* classed on the side of extortion.

1. Logre, *loc. cit.* (*Le Monde*, 30 Nov. 1948).

2. THE IMPENETRABLE FORTRESS

One should not see in this absolute respect for the freedom of the individual to confess or not, only an exaggeration of safeguards in favour of a suspect; nor should it be limited for fear of reducing justice to impotency. It is simply the application in law of a spiritual principle of an importance paramount to every other consideration, even to that of hampering justice. This is the principle of the inviolability of the conscience of every man, and the utter prohibition against breaking into this inner citadel by cozenage or guile.

It would in any case be the wrong moment for our judicial institutions to be altered on this point. Never has there been more pressing need to defend principles against impudent attempts to ignore them, which are a sign of our times. All kinds of practices are in existence which permit the violation of the mind and which give away the secrets of the soul to any inquisitor. The very 'climate' of life to-day is one in which the sense of the privacy of the personality tends to become lost: the lights in the streets, the headlines of the Press, the noises of the radio, the hallucinations of the cinema tend to draw the life of the inner consciousness outward until it is only skin deep. After the first shaking of the foundations of the spirit there comes infiltration by publicity slogans, by the obsession with commonplaces—and propaganda. All these continue the process of making man into a hollow puppet, void of all that is not a docile echo or a vague reflection of external values. Against such people inquisitions can play a fine game, for what secrecies has he left to defend? He is docile at making statements, filling forms, answering questions, making requests, swearing oaths. Soon he will, without a tremor, lend himself to public exercises in self-criticism, spontaneous admissions, mutual confessions: he will himself ask for the punishment deserved by those who have not conformed to doctrine or been faithful to the Party or loved their

Führer. When will this fanaticism for stripping the inner man stop?

All this arises from a general and serious evil: the loss of the sense of what is sacred. Respect for spiritual inwardness is only one form of the reverential awe which man should feel before certain principles which are beyond all argument, certain feelings one does not mock, certain things one does not attempt to rape. It is said to-day that this acceptance of limits to analysis and research, of the inviolability of mystery, is merely superstition and that it stands in the way of scientific advancement. Yet it must soon be realized that it is the basic rule by which human thought can be ordered, the only safeguard against a final lapse into insanity. There is no doubt that, as far as personal integrity is concerned, respect for the mystery of the soul is the only refuge, the final protection—nay, more, the sole guarantee that the soul itself shall continue to exist, whereas if it is to be opened up and improperly exteriorized, it is in actual peril of being destroyed.

It would be difficult to accept the contamination of justice by this tendency to dehumanize man, so that it forgets the respect due to the inwardness of the soul and lends itself to practices which are in effect a pitiless manhunt after forced confessions. It is utterly wrong to use technique to bring about by force the surrender of the secret self which it is unequivocally the privilege of each one to preserve. To accept such a barrier is indeed to accept a limit to the distance justice may be able to reach. But only those will deplore this who are tormented with a morbid and anxious judicial mind in which the desire for the protection of society is overshadowed by the pernicious will to dominate the individual and perhaps to hold him at their mercy. These perhaps will regret the inviolability of the secret soul, but others will recognize in it the humane side of justice as a social institution making claims to no greater right to penetrate another's conscience than is allowed in any other form of social relationship. *For in this sphere, minds com-*

municate only by signs. This general law does not allow man to have direct access to the conscience of another, the only minor exception being in the intimacies of love, while it is only entirely to be set aside in the contemplation of God. Any society or social institution claiming the right to infringe it would be committing a kind of sacrilege. Justice itself, however exalted its moral function, must agree that it must and can judge only by signs. For it is signs which a police interrogatory obtains, and medico-legal diagnosis is formed on signs. Every attempt at forceful penetration or direct influence on the mind is an extortion and risks taking judicial institutions back to the bad times of old, further aggravated by the power of modern technical methods.

Respect for the intimate self is a thing one has the right to expect from oneself as well as from others. That I am not completely transparent to myself is a psychological fact. It is also a demand for moral caution, for I am not likely to go scatheless if the depths of my being rise into my consciousness and upset the order of things in my mind which is the structure of my normal mental life. Light is required if one wants to explore an abyss and I can only safely get to know myself if I am enlightened by philosophy and helped by a moral code. If the self-examination which the West has practised for two thousand years has led to a surprising degree of deep understanding and subtlety, it is because it has always been guided by a sense of the need to build up morality at the same time as giving psychological self-knowledge. This desire for planned insight seems to have been replaced to-day by a love for plain catharsis, and the one who is tempted to make excursions into the darkness of his own being is further abetted by the change of guides. By an astounding tolerance in the laws governing medical practice, any unqualified charlatan may to-day call himself a psycho-analyst and provoke his patient to a lack of self-restraint which no other confidant or confessor would demand, and then practise on the naked *psyche* any dislocations of thought and feeling he may choose. We see as yet

THE SANCTITY OF SECRECY

only the indirect effects of this 'freedom', in the kind of literature in which the undisciplined mind is held triumphant. Its more secret ravages may soon come to light and its corrosive effects, under the guise of medicine, will have unbalanced the life of people, broken up families, made love into a neurosis—and filled the mental hospitals: all this as a result of having ignored the fact that self-penetration and analysis unguarded by the vigilance of superior controls results in nihilism.

I need scarcely draw attention to the notion that narcosis suggests to the minds of many practitioners an extension and a perfecting of this fantasmagoria of analysis. In the field of therapy it is for the conscience of the qualified practitioner to determine to what extent and under what safeguards the forcible lifting of inhibitions and conscious reticences should be allowed—and also for the conscience of the patient to decide, while in the full possession of his faculties, to what extent it is ethical for him to submit to it.

The limit to the use of such methods as a general measure in justice rests more clearly on the conscience of the one who might be called upon to be subjected to it. His refusal should be an argument against which there is no possible appeal, since it is not only the exercise of a right to protect his inner self, but it is more, since it is the performance of a duty never wilfully to give up his self-control.

Seen in this perspective, where secrecy becomes inviolable even by one who knows that secret, and where freewill can never properly be alienated, the last arguments in favour of medico-legal narcosis fail: it should never even be suggested to the accused as an option, nor made use of if he should consent to it. We have already seen what a contradiction it is in law to take it as a sign of guilt if a man refuses narcosis—a kind of blackmail which gives him freedom to refuse, then turns his use of that freedom against him. It would also be a moral error, for one has no right to make any judgment even of the reason behind such a refusal. It may indeed come from fear of giving oneself away, but it may arise also in an innocent person from a scruple, even a pride, in fulfilling the duty of keeping oneself always under control.

And let us make no false comparisons between the psychic and the bodily. For, admittedly, one gives up conscience and freedom in surgical anaesthesia. But this happens only incidentally to an operation on the body, and if, as sometimes happens, there are untimely confessions and revelations, they are accidental repercussions. But in narcosis, the removal of inhibitions is deliberate, the abandonment of self-control is an end which is being sought. There is even active assistance by the patient who answers questions put to him while his self-control is in suspense. This means that consent given by the patient at this moment has no value, since the consequences of self-abandonment cannot be foreseen. The subject cannot be certain that he will remain sufficiently lucid to stop making revelations at the point where he would wish—besides which, such confidences may reflect on other people.

For all these reasons the conclusion must be accepted, that narcosis is unacceptable in law and unjustified on moral grounds—and that by the conscience of the very person who might submit to it. For to submit would be to give illicit consent. Nobody has the right to take active part in suppressing his own power of self-determination, especially for operations which are uncontrollable and the course of which is not to be predicted and which result directly from that very act of self-suppression.

Thus consent by the accused has no valid sanction for the expert. True, such consent might, from one angle, save the accused trouble, but it is void in law and unethical on the moral plane.

People may say this is all too subtle. But it is out of subtleties that civilization is built. Some people accept medico-legal narcosis with a light-heartedness which shows that specialization in science and a prejudice in favour of

THE SANCTITY OF SECRECY

technology have fogged their minds to the sense of spiritual realities. Let me add that the Christian, more than any other, has to be on his guard, since his very religion recognizes and hallows the sacred character of confession and of secrecy.

Above the mystery of the soul, Christianity places the overshadowing mystery of God: two unknowables which can only be resolved when man comes to see 'face to face'. Yet one of these, in the partial light of life down here, is like a guarantee and a safeguard of the other. The insight of God into the depths of a soul is beyond our comprehension. But it shows the mockery and the sacrilege of human ambition trying to usurp a like power of penetration. To a Christian, respect for the secrecy of the soul is the same thing as the respect of the power over that soul which belongs to God alone.

This is why the Catholic Church has marked the confessional with a sacramental seal. It was not enough to regard an act of self-knowledge through confession as promising a power of subjective ordering and reconstruction —in which the Church followed the intuitions of Socratic wisdom clarified and focused in the light of moral theology. It went further, and by sanctifying and thereby preserving the ability to confess freely, it placed confession under the protection of God, and thereby refused the confessor any human rights to use it for inquisitorial purposes. The obligation laid on the confessor is to maintain such absolute discretion that it amounts to complete prohibition. Apart from invoking the help of God, he is not even allowed to *think* about a confession after it has been received. This shows clearly that absolute and unreserved confession is only possible when the power of one man over another is no longer allowed to exist.

Here is the supreme spiritual justification of the judicial principle governing free confession. The judge may have direct cognizance of it, or it may be that it comes to him only as an echo from the depths of himself, arising from a spiritual civilization steeped in Christianity; but if he respects the impenetrability of the freedom of the heart, he is obeying a basic intuition which is infinitely delicate and infinitely precious. It shows the feeling that human justice has certain limits, and that if it tries to go beyond these limits it takes to itself a right to total invasion of the soul which belongs only to God, and lays claim to an abominable dominion of man over other men. It is only before God that there is no right to deny the truth. But this absolute openness is one which no human judge can obtain otherwise than by an act of violence to the self.

Here is the core of the problem. The use of pentothal, the abuses which may arise from it, the pretension of man to explore the conscience of others, the forcible rape of secrecy, are a diabolical parody of the all-seeingness of God.

Chapter 8

BACKGROUND

IT may seem that we have wandered far from our subject. In reality we are directly on it. Pentothal is all the more to be feared in that it has come into a world in process of spiritual disintegration. The question of its use is identical with that of the safety of man in a dehumanized civilization.

No doubt, as we have shown, this drug carries its own intrinsic dangers, its essential perversity. But if we admit that in the hands of some people it may be both safe and valuable, what are the things which can make it so? There should be a code of safeguards which could act as a firm rampart against all abuses: a free community, a healthy justice, independence of medical practice.

But these codes lie in pieces. It is folly or blindness to argue as if they still held firm, and to try and resolve the problem of pentothal in terms of the pulpit or the laboratory. We are concerned with forensic medicine in a world already given over to power politics, to judicial systems which degrade. Inevitably, under these conditions, pentothal must become, if it is not already, one of a number of means open to the use of tyranny, whose claims are always increasing and whose methods, when exasperated, turn to pure savagery.

1. POLITICAL

Some readers may have thought that the foregoing pages contain nothing more than finicky arguments about a problem which, when all is said and done, concerns criminals often dangerous, sometimes irredeemable. The medico-legal expert and the judge now have to work at a human level where all the subtleties of freedom as to confession, and respect for secrecy are practically meaningless. Yet even at this level we see only part of the picture. In the methods it uses, justice itself stands at the bar. Its own dignity is in question even more than the rights of those it has to try. The matter cannot rest at this point. The problem of respect for the accused goes a long way further than the limits of consideration for a criminal, and in many cases and in many countries in differing degrees, judicial procedure has virtually become a means of exterminating innocent people. The safeguards given by the code of criminal investigation—the code of honest people—have never been more precious than they are to-day, when so many honest people are dragged before the judges. One sees judicial institutions seized upon by states which enslave them, and rot them by tainting them with political ideas and the insistence on efficacy. They are thereby turned away from checking crime and used simply to reduce opposition. These justices attack the conscience of its victims, and especially those of quiet people with a moral standard which furnishes no excuse for such ferocity.

It is thus all the more urgent that the innocent be defended against false justice. For it is now not only a matter of protecting him against ordinary miscarriages of justice—frequent enough, but unwitting—which are the consequences of the weakness and stupidity of men. We are dealing with a whole legion of innocent people already forced into submission, already caught in systematized miscarriages by a justice made fanatical and built up by politicians into a relentless killing machine.

The political phenomenon of the degradation of justice makes pentothal all the more important. For the sake of the innocent, superior principles of legal procedure, such as our own, must be at all costs defended, and that, even at the cost of allowing a few undeserved loopholes to authentic criminals.

The same consideration of political climate should make us repudiate the final argument of the partisans of pentothal. That is the argument about social security. There are cases, we are told, where, in self-defence against evil-doers, '*society has the right to know*',[1] and the exceptional methods used for showing up evil intentions try to justify themselves by consideration of the collective good. '*Do not the interests of society take precedence over respect for individual freedom?*'[2] It is time we forgot these down-at-heel platitudes, dubious in themselves, and liable to serve as a pretext for the worst of undertakings.

The alleged opposition between the good of society and individual freedom is inconsistent, and the question of pentothal cannot be summarized as one of alternatives between the two, in which the choice of either might be called sentimental.[3] My opposition arises, not from a demoded attachment to fusty romanticism about liberty, or to a kind of anarchic individualism. The problem of pentothal is not one of individual versus society, but one of ends and means. We have to decide whether it is permissible to defend society by using means which are contrary to the moral and spiritual ideals which make life in that society worth while, and which are the cement which hold it together. In a group where the common weal is felt and loved otherwise than as the crushing weight of the collective on the individual, social security is directly governed by respect for individual freedom. We know also that nothing is more lethal to social unity than distorted justice, for its proceedings cause fear, rebellion and hatred. In pretending to defend the common good it actually destroys the

1. Lebret: *op. cit.* (*Ann. de méd. lég.*, March–April 1949, p. 59). '*Others believe that in the presence of a criminal, society has to defend itself as best it can,*' crudely says another expert (Charlin, *op. cit., Ann. de méd. lég.*, July–Aug. 1949, p. 170).

2. Trillot: *op. cit.* (*Acta med. leg. et soc.*, Brussels, 1949, p. 651).

3. Trillot: *op. cit.*, '*The medico-legal expert must do away with all sentimental considerations in the general interest*' (*Ann. de méd. lég.*, July–Aug. 1949, p. 170).

communion of mind with mind. Justice in a civilized society can only defend common interests through its respect for the freedom of the person. Thus the dilemma suggested is not a real one, and pentothal is not to be disposed of in terms of it.

It is indeed strange to have to consider arguments on the need to defend honest people against evil-doers at a time when it is so obvious that the greatest dangers arise from the evil forms of that very justice. In the interest of society, it is clear that the good must be defended against the wicked; but it is equally clear that the good should be protected against being themselves labelled wicked. How many honourable citizens have ever had to fight a criminal? I personally know far more people who have suffered when they have had to fight against the Law. God preserve me from the judges! I had far rather deal directly, myself, with any criminal!

Moreover, we are not even told what is this 'Society', which stands in such need of protection, which 'has the right to know'. Entities whose names are written with capitals are usually fictitious; and, in this case, pregnant with menace. For even in a stable society, those who speak in the name of 'Society' thereby scarcely acquire infallibility, nor the right to do what they like. This is all the more so in circumstances where the claim to represent 'Society' is no more than a feeble excuse for trying to dominate. It only remains for those in power to decide, in the name of 'Society', that everybody who disagrees with them is a traitor, a criminal—and that they therefore have the unlimited 'right to know'.

There is a political slant, therefore, in my fear of the police use of pentothal. Those who try to reassure us by saying that narcosis is a scientific method needing care and practice, and that it neither can nor must become a part of police procedure, are strangely blind to the practical aspects of the question. It is a forlorn and theoretical hope that the police will never act otherwise than as subordinates of the judiciary, conform to its principles and abide by its rules and customs. They will never agree to account to the Court for every step taken, every detail of the methods used, and so ensure that they have not trespassed on the judicial field.

The source of police improprieties such as are at last stirring the public conscience, is in the tendency for the police to trespass on the judicial rôle, as for instance by cross-examination of the accused. The judges themselves have tacitly connived at this, allowing the police to use dirty methods which they themselves would consider it beneath their dignity to use openly. Several scandalous cases have been brought to light, showing the brutality and the mistakes which arise from independent police action— so much so that the name of justice itself has been tarnished to the extent that the judges have at last become aware of the danger to themselves. They have begun to distrust the police and hence, indirectly, to resume their authority, thereby pointing out the subordinate rôle of the police officer. The whole cause of police abuses is there. We need seek no further. Moreover, since the Bench allowed them to come into being, it can also abolish them by rebuilding a proper hierarchical order in place of the one which has been upset, and regaining the authority they have allowed others to usurp.

If, then, police abuses are due to police independence, there are cases where they cannot be stopped. That is the case where the police is not responsible to higher judicial authority. The counter-espionage service known as that of National Security is such a case, and it is here that the worst horrors are to be found. There are also other police forces run by governments, and responsible, not to judges but to politicians who are ready to use any means which will keep them in power and who, in turn, are responsible to nobody else. This has happened in France, and there is no guarantee that we shall not see it again. Those who advocate the use of pentothal argue as if we were secure in never having any truck with a police which was not ideally submissive to the spirit of judicial authority. If this were true, one might then feel sure that only medical experts would use this tricky drug for proper purposes and that the police would be debarred from doing so. But there can be no such security when one has to do with thugs in the pay of powers whose sole aim is to hunt down and destroy those it does not like.

I foresee an objection: that is that, under such conditions as I have suggested, no amount of prohibition, whether absolute or complete, would hold good ; hence we are wasting our time. True: oppositions and protests would vanish like straws in the wind, were there to be a universal extension of political régimes which use the Law as a means of extermination. Yet that is not reason enough for silence, and even if the protest were eventually to be ignored, one might be accused of complicity, since evil can only triumph when prior consent opens the way for it, that is when the minds of the very people concerned with keeping it at bay have been led to accept and favour it. Those who, in any capacity whatever, have a responsibility for the preservation of spiritual values must not give a bad example by agreeing, even tacitly, to abuses. Their protests may do no more, but they will have prevented the establishment of a precedent, and so will have helped to add to the resistance in the minds of the people towards accepting them. In this way, no unscrupulous policeman will be able to claim to be acting according to precedent, and hence as the agent of true justice, while he will on the contrary be likely to hit up against a positive body of adverse opinion.

The *duty to prohibit*, which belongs to the protestor, must not be side-tracked in favour of another pretext. It may be said that the effort to avoid *potential* mistakes in the use of pentothal is to tilt at windmills and to forget the real foe. For the police already effectively use means of constraint far more brutal and grave, and which are real tortures. These, it will be said, should be the first object of attack,[1]

1. Mellor: *La Torture*, p. 317, supported by further correspondence with the author.

while the battle against pentothal is against a hypothesis, not a fact. It is surely more important to protect a suspect against police officers who, acting *in camera*, break his limbs and skull at their leisure, than against the use of narcosis which has never yet taken place. This, however, burkes the issue: both battles are really one, and attack a single evil. The campaign for abolition must cover all forms of torture, whether overt or concealed. And we have already seen that narcosis belongs to the spirit of torture and is even more insidious than the infliction of bodily pain. One must not reintroduce by one door practices which have been already dismissed by another. It is easy enough to deal with the principles of private police interrogation, far more difficult to combat similar compulsive methods when introduced by the solemn practices of justice, even when camouflaged under the authority of science.

No single loophole must be overlooked. The battle is one, and it is against a threat to our civilization. However different modern techniques may be from those of the past, the background is the same, that is, a desire for improper power to dominate and exploit mankind even if this means also to destroy it; and that by means which should be used only for its good. The evil is clearly political, since political power is to-day the tool of barbarism. Behind every technique of power stands the monstrous shadow of the State— if a body which has lost its traditions and is often only a power captured by chance by a band of greedy, ambitious people, can be so called—an aggressive power, making capital out of every technical means which will add to its grip on the community. There is for instance nothing to fear from atomic energy other than its use by imperialistic, economic or military ideologists worse than any ever known to history. The same applies to means of communication, to broadcasting, unless used by a tyranny for propaganda and spiritual hoodwinking based on lies. Even productive technique has become a degradation of work, where the capitalist state has connived at enslaving the worker by

State Socialism and Marxist economics. Finally, pharmacy and psychiatry are only dangerous when they are used outside the medical sphere, in such ways as they have already been used by political powers, to get the minds of people at their mercy and to abolish all resistance. If modern scientific technique has in fact become the technique of prostitution, it is simply because it has fallen into the hands of states which rule by debasing. Scientific barbarism is due to political barbarism.

Any attempt to enlarge the sphere of the use of pentothal by bringing it into the field of justice may go still further and reach the realm of politics. This fear might be deemed vain, were it not for the Cens case, which was surely a matter of politics. There was also the case of the relentless pursuit of the Belgian. In each of these, scientific technique was degraded through what may have been unconscious vindictiveness, into a political technique in the game of 'hunt the traitor'.

The prime virtue of a medical expert is to have no party views, a difficult matter where 'politism' and its fanaticism come into play. If civilization were functioning normally, we might feel reasonably sure that justice would not persecute the criminal, because the peace of mind of both judge and expert would be undisturbed, and there would be no risk of means of investigation being used for political purposes of extortion. But we are in a state of political barbarism. Hence the opposition to pentothal, in so far as it is also an opposition to the misuse of science for political ends, is part of the complex political situation of the times. It is not to be reduced, except by complete stultification, to a simple matter of forensic medicine, and the more difficult the problem, the more seriously it needs to be taken. The circumstances which would normally safeguard us are far from secure, and this makes it all the more imperative that pentothal should be kept within the walls of hospitals and clinics, not launched into a world only too ready to use it to debase mankind. And should political barbarism ever triumph, let us not be guilty of having prepared the place for abuses by tacit consent. On the contrary, let the horror we have constantly felt on the subject be the last line of resistance as well, perhaps, as giving us the last strength to refuse it.

2. JUSTICE IN DOUBT

The danger would be small, were it contained and rectified by solid medical and legal codes. But there are many deficiencies in these which ruin any hope of safety. Neither justice nor medicine has preserved its independence from the encroachments of politics. Hence for justice to allow itself to use techniques of so delicate a nature for mental *expertise* requires both that it shall never be used improperly by the police, and that justice should be entirely divorced from politics. This is not the case to-day in many countries.

There is no need to emphasize the need for justice to be independent of the State. We no longer live in an age when Parliament was in constant and vigorous rebellion against royal authority. Since the day when the authority of the State was separated from that of justice, the latter has tended to become subservient to contradictory forces. We need pass no moral judgment on this fact, but it is evident that justice is no longer in a position to stand firm against the possible use of narcosis for political ends: at best it would offer only a feeble resistance to the demands of the State, and we can have no faith that it would ensure only its proper use.

We have already seen how weak is the control which the Law has over the police, how judges have become accomplices in horrors and brutal treatment by allowing prisoners to be brought into Court in frightful physical condition, and in failing to take action to protect them. If this is already so, how can one hope that pentothal will never be misused by the police as a 'truth serum'?

Still more serious is the question of the vast and soulless bureaucracy which lives entrenched behind piles of papers, bent on covering itself in every direction, as slow and uncertain in its actions as the most inhuman administrative machine. The result—as we saw in the Cens case—was the most abominable abuses, due to prolongation of detention before trial. Prisoners have sometimes waited months or even years before anybody paid any attention to them. After as much as four years in gaol, they have even been found not guilty. People have been 'forgotten' in prison, because their files had been mislaid, and often, arrest and detention have been carried out entirely unnecessarily and unjustifiably, without the prosecution bringing any charge against the victim.[1] Such things show so scant an attention to possible innocence, so callous an indifference to suffering, so great a disrespect for humanity, that no honest man is safe. One cannot have faith in a system where nobody is responsible, and against which the only safeguard lies in a justice based on principles which have been lost.

Justice, as we have said, is in a critical state, and if some of the projected reforms seem bent on increasing our safeguards, others tend equally to abrogate basic principles—recommendations for the use of pentothal among them. This shows that the advocates of these reforms wish to deepen the work of the medical expert, and thereby to transform the whole pattern of justice. Some advocate the right of the medical expert to keep secrecy—a thing we have already shown to be untenable—but are willing to upset the whole nature of a trial to satisfy the passion of a few doctors for a new toy. Another proposition comes, this time from a jurist.[2] It is to generalize the use of pentothal in a penal

1. Annotation in *Le Monde*, 9 July, 1948.
2. At Lourdes, in 1948, the Chaplain of the prison of Fresnes reminded us that 350 political prisoners still awaited trial after five years of detention. Worse still, detention before capital punishment, shackled with weights, '*thirty condemned people are awaiting execution in Fresnes, one, a woman, for over nine months*'.

[And, more recently, we have had the trial of those accused of the Oradour massacre, after some eight years.—*Tr.*]

system where indeterminate sentences would be used. '*When one is using fairly modern principles, deprivation of liberty tends to become more or less indeterminate.*' Liberation is then made conditional on psychiatric tests. We are told here that narcosis can, in such an event, only act in favour of the prisoner or, at worst, be neutral to him, since it would '*not order a sentence, but study the possibility of terminating it*'. But if so, we should know more of this principle of the indeterminate sentence, for if it refers to a penalty with a prefixed maximum, and it becomes a matter of setting the prisoner free before the end of that term, all is well. It would mean that justice and medicine were surrounding the prisoner with humane attentions, not treating him as an outcast, and would agree with the principles advocated by Professors Richet and Desoille as a reform of the penal system. Pentothal might safely be used in such a case. But if the principle of indeterminacy means that not even a maximum term is fixed, the liberation of the prisoner would depend entirely on medical recommendations—and one's worst fears would be justified.

Two judicial guarantees are required if imprisonment is not to be odious and barbaric: a man in prison has the right to know, (1) why he is there, and (2) when he is to be released. It would be moral torture to leave a prisoner in doubt as to the day and even the eventual possibility of his liberation. And when it comes to political powers, one shudders to think what use might be made of indeterminate sentences, under the pretext of social re-education, until the gaolers could certify that the prisoner had repented of his freely held views.

Further, such a measure would extend to absurd lengths the 'imperialism' of the medico-legal expert. Medical reports already carry far too much weight in judicial decisions, and often decide the fate of the accused. Are doctors then to become the ultimate arbiters of justice?

One of the most significant points in the crisis of uncertainty which seems to be afflicting justice to-day is that it does not see where it stands in relation to science. Clearly, it should retain its primacy and its authority, but it should also use as much science as it requires. The difficulty, however, is not due to 'progress' in the technique of mental investigation, but to the inability of justice to determine how much science can be allowed to have its say, and where it should be kept quiet. A recent affair at the Assizes at Riom shows this in a very sad case. The head of an 'aerium' was found dead in the room of a member of the staff who was his mistress. The local doctor certified death from natural causes, that is, from cerebral haemorrhage. The police, however, questioned the staff of the institution and, after interrogations, one of which lasted twenty-eight consecutive hours, induced two of the women staff to 'confess' to murder—after which, for some reason unstated, only one of the confessions was treated as genuine. The body was exhumed and it was indeed found that there was a clot of blood in the brain, but some experts said it was recent, and had caused death, others that it was an old one and had not caused death. There were also marks on the neck which some said pointed to strangulation, while others said they were secondary to the cerebral haemorrhage. The case revealed both the forcible methods used by the police and the disagreement of the doctors; hence, the valuelessness of the alleged confessions obtained by the former, and the doubts among the latter. There was shown to be complete absence of motive. The accused was acquitted—but only after thirteen months in prison.

The drama was in three acts:

1. With the police: This should have been the time, now or never, to use scientific technique in collecting evidence. But no: they simply leaped on suspects and tried to force a confession: the laboratory was replaced by the torture chamber. Meanwhile, the deceased was buried only to be exhumed after the body had been in the ground far too long either to be pleasant or to afford clear evidence of the mode of death. Science was not used while time was in its favour,

and outrageous and untimely means were used both on the wrong people and by those who had no business to use them.

2. Medical: It was too late, as we have seen, for science to prove effective. Moreover, the case was fogged by a false confession already obtained. Medicine, not being an exact science, moreover, expert contradicted expert, not so much on scientific grounds as on grounds of their prejudice for or against the truth of the confession of guilt. The confusion already started by the police was thus doubled.

3. Judicial: Set off by the police, bogged down by the doctors, justice could scarcely act objectively. The Court case started by a disquisition against torture, followed by a medical dispute. Twelve sensible Auvergnats, seeing this, sent the lot of them about their business, the Bench acting simply as spectators. Had the latter had to cope with the case without a jury (and I hold no brief for 'popular' justice) I do not know what their verdict might have been. And the Public Prosecutor, pleading anyway in a void, admitted there were extenuating circumstances! This was the last straw! Extenuating what?

True, justice did not miscarry in this case. But it was a near-miss and perhaps more instructive than if miscarriage had actually taken place. Let us also remember that a woman's life was in peril, and that she suffered thirteen months' detention as a result of this medico-legal-police imbroglio. The only thing lacking was pentothal, and even that came into sight and was only avoided because its use depended on a doctor who, fortunately, did not hold the superstition, and so saved justice from yet another motive for losing its head.

Why the imbroglio? Because justice had failed to put each thing in its place and lacked certain essential principles, that is, those which would define the proper rôle of the police, the weight to be given to medical opinion, the importance of moral elements (in this case abundantly clear, since there was neither psychological nor moral motive for the crime). The lack of assertion of the primacy of the judge on the Bench over police or medical acts is the basic cause of all this.

One has to ask oneself whether a new source of data requiring to be very carefully studied and understood, can safely be brought into play before a justice which has ceased to try and study or understand. And, moreover, is it safe to bring pseudo-scientific superstition to bear on a justice which is so unsure of itself?

3. OVER-CONFIDENT MEDICINE

Justice having lost its faith in itself, medicine has gained too much. The effects are the same, the reasons also, though in reverse, and medicine gives us no guarantees against the abuse of pentothal.

Let me say again that I am attacking no individual nor any corporate body. Neither justice nor medicine is on trial: since the days of Rabelais and Molière, such subjects are no longer original and, moreover, are not the purpose of my essay. We are examining a social situation and in the complexity of this both professions are inseparable and, moreover, are in process of dangerous transformations. One may think what one likes about these: I do not want to discuss them, being no social reformer, and I am quite willing to leave it to those whose job it is to try and restore the status of either the judicial or the medical profession. Yet I have the right to feel anxious over such transformations—deformations, rather—when they lead to the introduction of a novelty the risks of which could only be exorcized by the professional bodies responsible for its use if they themselves were entirely healthy.

In this century of unbelief, we are dominated by a superstition: that of belief in science and technology. These terms are allowed so wide an application that they include courses of action which are neither science nor art, and which are not properly techniques. Yet out of ignorance we accept that they have virtues of safety and efficacy which they have not. This is the position of medicine.

Such an atmosphere may infect even people well placed not to be taken in. If incense is burned before a person for a long time, there is always the risk that he may eventually come to believe that he really is something of a god. In a world where the technician is king, the physician becomes a god and so tends to lose sight of the true meaning and the human quality of his art. The legitimate confidence which the doctor should inspire as a man is unconsciously allowed to reflect into the science he practises: the genuine virtues of the doctor himself are the very things which give false value to medicine itself. The authority given him by his place in society and in administration is sometimes very valuable in troubled times when rations, leave, exemptions from service and the like, depend on his opinion. But it makes it too easy for him to identify himself, the man, with the authority which he represents as an agent of science, and hence also to acquire a false belief in the absolute scientific value of medicine. I will not enlarge on Alain's vilification of 'the little tyrant', but what I want to say is that when a man finds himself clothed in such authority, it is humanly impossible for him not to believe that he has become the high-priest of an exact science. In the most difficult circumstance of his professional life, the doctor has perforce to safeguard himself against destructive criticism by taking up a highly defensive attitude. Few people will allow him the right to say that he does not know, and it is anyway his task to try and inspire confidence in those around him even when he feels himself in doubt. He is always expected to act and behave as if he did know. There are doubtless some who can carry the responsibility of their terrible profession without illusions; but most fall into the error of thinking that the demand that they make a decision is identical with being sure of exactly what they are about to do.

All this, moreover, is happening in a scientific climate which is highly active, and where the taste for novelty inspires unlimited faith in research. This helps to raise in the minds of the very ones who most need to remain objective, an implicit and often unconscious superstition as regards the scientific nature of medicine. This bad example is set from on high, where there is a pontificate which allows neither resistance nor contradiction. Sick people are docile, so are pupils: hence science becomes irresistible. This may indeed become dangerous, and would have done so in the case just cited, had it not been for the greater modesty and caution of those who remembered the wise saying that *'in medicine one should not be unduly positive'*. For here a learned professor might have forfeited the life of an innocent woman on the slight yet authoritative statements he had made.

It should be pointed out moreover that these contradicted the teachings he himself gave in his lectures. For, as a teacher, he said that *'effusions in the carotid region may follow on cerebral hæmorrhage'*, while, as a medical expert, he said that the marks in this case were evidence of strangulation, despite the post-mortem findings of cerebral haemorrhage. In the Cens case, too, another learned expert was so confident of his results (he contradicted himself afterwards) that he affirmed that *'Cens was cured'*.[1] What unshakable faith we should have in science after these demonstrations!

Fortunately, there are other teachers whose knowledge is coupled with discretion. One of the most competent unhesitatingly stated the exacting and delicate conditions under which alone narco-analysis should be practised, so that *'it should not run the risk of becoming a menace in the hands of physicians as incompetent as they are inexperienced.'*[2] Indeed, the very spirit of science consists in a superior use of scientific doubt and moral caution. Lack of these virtues

1. Heuyer and Favreau (*Ann. de méd. lég.*, Mar.–April 1948, p. 102).
2. Cornil and Ollivier, *Problèmes de sélection et d'actualités médico-sociales*, p. 146.

makes the use of pentothal a risky game, and should its use become general, one must hope also that it will be saved from improper use by an equally general growth of qualities already scarce enough and which, in the atmosphere of the present day, are likely to become still more so.

Other grounds for suspicion are to be found in the bad tendency, which is always gaining ground, for medicine to be run by the government. Bureaucracy and medicine tend to become ever more closely mingled, though it is not clear whether it is a case of the State using medicine in order to strengthen its hold on the people, or medicine exploiting the State to increase its own power. Doctors strongly object to red tape, yet it is through their own initiative that herd medicine is being promoted. This is strangely inconsistent, for if doctors do not themselves want to be regimented, they should not lend themselves to the regimentation of their patients. It is claimed that the State should govern every moment of a man's life, from conception to burial on the— so far dubious—plea of the scientific organization of public health. This dream of compulsory medicine and therapy through statistics is no more than the ideal of modern collectivism dressed in scientific garb—i.e., the complete documenting of the whole of mankind.

This is a terrifying phenomenon of scientific authoritarianism. The pursuit of science has, by deterioration and over-diffusion, changed its character from a philosophical idea to a means of political tyranny. In the name of Science, the State is going to manage everything and everybody; and medicine, the science of man himself, is the most potent of its instruments for dominating man. One can no longer say that this strange wedding of scientists and tyrants, of which Renan wrote a fantastic story, is not haunting the dreams of many people. An example of how scientific idolatry, apparently harmless, can change, even among the best people, into a fearful appetite for political power, is to be found in the curious pages where Dr. Carrel foresees the rôle which medicine, the super-science, should play in government. He suggests that the State of the future, a reincarnation of enlightened despotism, will become embodied in the person of some dictator, surrounded by scientific counsellors.[1]

This kind of tyranny can and anyway does exist already without a dictator: democracy plays the part well enough. The Parliamentary Commission on Public Health (in France) of which the chairman was, I believe, a doctor, has imposed on us in an instant, the compulsory use of B.C.G.,[2] and that, despite all uncertainties about it, disregarding all protests, without consultation with learned societies, public discussion or parliamentary debate. Why? Because that is science: these gentlemen are scientists, so the herd must submit in silence. Members of Parliament, who are usually far from silent, fell for this and voted as one man: clearly, parliamentary control must play second fiddle to medical dictatorship. Technocracy is the most odious of dictatorships, for it claims, in the name of Science, to have to render no accounts—and everybody thinks this is quite as it should be.

I shall soon be able to take no step in life, to marry, to make love, to send my children to school, to take a job, travel, eat, drink, without a medical certificate. Only pentothal is needed to complete enslavement to the State through medicine. In the best-of-all-worlds-to-be, the Great Tyrant will know how to use his medical Gestapo: I shall soon no longer be allowed to vote, to make my tax

1. Alexis Carrel, *L'Homme cet Inconnu*, p. 353 (Plon, Paris, 1941). (There is an English translation of this, under the title, *Man the Unknown*, recently reprinted in the Pelican edition.—*Tr.*) See also the whole of the last chapter of this book, and *Cahiers de la Fondation Française pour l'étude des problèmes humains*, No. 1, 1943. It is only fair, however, to distinguish between the attitude of Carrel and the arrogant and limited one of Marxist materialism.

2. B.C.G.: A vaccine used to immunize against tuberculosis.—*Tr.*

BACKGROUND

returns, to join the Party, to 'go sick' under the National Health Insurance, to have an identity card or a ration book unless I produce a certificate of loyalty and docility, proved under barbiturate narcosis.

To sum up: there would be the greatest risk, were pentothal to be introduced into forensic medicine, lest it be used by the police for political ends. If this should happen, there would be no appeal to either of the two great institutions which should protect the freedom of the individual against arbitrary violence. Justice is too unsure of itself, too much subservient to the State. Medicine is too cocksure and, being on good terms with the State, would not defend us against her friend. Pentothal would run wild as soon as the first door to it was opened, and nothing could henceforth prevent the worst abuse of it. These are the reasons behind the automatic recoil which many people feel from pentothal, and these are the prospects which use of the drug in the precarious state of our civilization suggest to anybody at all clear-sighted.

4. JUSTICE BY DEGRADATION

The world of debased politics is not merely potential, it exists already in all its hideousness. We need only look there to see what takes place when justice is ruled by politics.

It may be said that totalitarian trials have nothing to do with pentothal, and that it does not explain the Moscow purges of 1937, nor the more recent affairs in countries where the proletariat is said to dictate. Moreover, it may be argued that these are simply cases of persecution of religion—as in the cases of Bishop Stepinaç, Cardinal Mindszenty, the Pastors of Sofia, and the Jesuits of Lubljana —or else a settling of accounts between people in power —as in the cases of Petkov, Rajk, and Kostov—so that, by quoting them, we are only giving way to unfounded anxiety.

These trials, we are told, have led the public to believe that the strange confessions and repudiations of faith made by the accused were due to the action of a drug. It may be well to clarify matters.

If we are puzzled as to the means used in Communist persecution to make the accused confess their guilt, this is because of the complete incongruity between what was known of them in their normal state and how they behaved in Court. Where politics are concerned, it is possible to attribute the extravagance of almost delirious self-accusation to the temperament of the Slav, or to a kind of logic of self-destruction which, Koestler suggests, is part of the Marxist mentality. But when it comes to anti-Christian trials, no explanation in terms of normal psychology— assuming any of those cited to have been normal—is tenable. There is too complete a contradiction between the accused as they were, and what they have become. Their admissions are entirely out of gear with their character, their previous actions, all their antecedents. Moreover, the same scenario is repeated so exactly in each case, that only one explanation is possible, that is, the transformation of the personality by violent means. From this there arises the hypothesis of a diabolic drug, able to disintegrate the will and to inoculate into the mind of a man who has been reduced to the state of a living corpse, the theme which leads him to seek his own perdition.

History may answer the enigma, for the moment we can only speculate. We have no direct proof that drugs were used on the Primate of Hungary. The rumours and the newspaper articles which said so were premature and ill-informed. We simply do not know, though we may make conjectures from the physico-chemical angle. But they are no more than conjectures, however permissible and plausible.

The question is whether there is any drug known to Western science which is capable of bringing about an entire transformation of the personality. Nobody can be entirely positive, but some think it possible. One thing however is certain: it is not pentothal, since, even though this can extort statements while the personality is altered by it, the alteration is only transitory and does not produce this kind of psychic *volte-face*. Pentothal may even have an opposite result, for everything in these cases shows, not that the victim suffers from inhibition of control, such as barbiturates produce, together with euphoria, but rather a positive tension of anxiety which urges them on to make purely voluntary confessions. Only a lasting state of anxiety seems to account for the condition of the accused, and published photographs confirm this by showing the characteristic expression of anguish on their faces. *To cause anxiety:* this is the secret of the torturer. Drugs may be used, but only along with physical torments.[1]

It is possible [writes a psychiatrist] that amphetamine bodies are used, maxiton being the most powerful, in high doses and under specially arranged conditions, such as when the victim is compelled to stand up for from four to eight days—which would be impossible without artificial doping. The anxiety set off in this way and increased by physiological breakdown (maxiton makes people lose weight, burn up quicker, brings about partial inanition and insomnia) would be followed up by suggestions of the nature of the guilt to be admitted: whence the tone of sincerity and conviction in the self-accusation of the victim.

There can be no doubt that sovietized police forces have a technique of mental disintegration which is horribly efficient. Hunger, thirst, sleeplessness; darkness or dazzling light; psychological tortures by vertigo, hallucination, frenzy; threats and monstrous blackmail; drug intoxication: all of these may be used, separately or together. They know literally how to abolish the personality, to cause complete deflation so that the tortured mind stands empty of everything except an anguish next door to madness. His private

1. See p. 32, and the notes on the effect of the amphetamines in causing 'discharge of anxiety'.

convictions and freewill are deleted. Then, catching hold of any positive suggestion, like a drowning man clutching at the first piece of wreckage which comes his way, he accepts the themes inoculated into him in the interrogation, and these acquire a hallucinatory power of self-conviction.

Pentothal may seem a harmless anodine alongside this. I agree, while pointing out that a dangerous practice is not justified by being less bad than another. But we have to consider not only the intrinsic properties of particular drugs, nor the fact that they may be used, so much as the attitude of mind common to all these things, that is, the determination to extort admissions, to debase the victim, to destroy his mind and dislocate his will, towards which the mildness of pentothal is only the first step. The amphetamines are the second.

Such is the problem. In looking at the background of totalitarian actions, we are not looking only at a bogy, but considering an actual situation. It may have nothing directly to do with pentothal, but it shows how easily justice may become expert at suborning the mind. Pentothal may be only small beer in this, but it nevertheless fits well into the code of procedure and, as such, is quite enough to inspire us with horror.

Justice becomes identified with revolutionary movements when it feels itself to be part of historical trends and sets to work to eliminate opposition and resistance on the grounds that these impede the currents of life which are moving into the future. Such is totalitarian justice to-day, and it sets out systematically to do away with those who disagree with it, and do so with unappeasable fanaticism. The definition of guilt becomes indefinitely extended, innocence is entirely disregarded. More, sincerity and guiltlessness in an opponent are even looked upon as aggravating circumstances. The sole criterion of what is just is what is politically efficacious.

All this rests on a stupid notion that *purification* is a possible achievement, that all variety of opinion save one can be got rid of, so that unanimity becomes as much a fact as purity of a chemical substance. This must logically lead the purifier to total extermination. '*We will turn the whole of France into a cemetery rather than fail to regenerate her after our own desire,*' said Saint Just. '*Purification is not complete,*' they say to-day. And naturally so, since it can never be achieved so long as one free man survives together with the purifier. The result is complete self-destruction. In the ferocity of purification, the Terror scheduled endless gradations of guilt. There were 'enemies of the People', 'suspects', 'believed suspects', while innocence itself was only considered as potential guilt. Normal justice seeks for the guilty among a mass of innocent people, revolutionary justice suspects the mass and tries to find the 'pure' among them.

So the first step is to imprison everybody: '*Too many guilty people would escape if one did not arrest the innocent,*' says Carrier. '*Better the death of an innocent man than a spy at liberty,*' recently said M. Claude Bonnet. After this, bit by bit, one releases those who pass muster. It does not matter how long this takes, provided it is done, nor how many innocent people are persecuted provided possibly guilty people are held. In revolutionary justice, imprisonment prior to trial is the permanent state of every citizen.

All revolutionary purges, moreover, attack freedom of thought, and an honest journalist is a greater danger than one who is not. '*The more intellectually honest a politician may be, the more responsible and guilty he is in my eyes: he is a serious political adversary,*' wrote M. David Rousset. This is as good a definition as possible of a justice in which roguery is an attenuating factor: one may always make a rogue into an ally.

Yet even worse than suppression of freedom and truth is the tendency of revolutionary justice to degrade man. They are not content to kill outright, they must first extract a confession, then smirch the victim's name for the sake of their own propaganda. Why trouble about confession? Doubtless from fanaticism: there is no worse violator of others than a frenzied politician. Conformity of action is not enough, there must also be conformity of thought, and that final act of submission which occurs when a rebel confesses his guilt. Further, it justifies his acts. He does not require confession to strengthen the conviction of the judge and to satisfy his conscience (such things belong to another kind of justice) but as a pretext for ferocity and for using the pitiless killing machine. In short, it is pure sadism. The totalitarian judge, like the politician who uses him, demands that the accused should be entirely delivered over to him. Only one form of defence is allowed: admission of guilt and a plea for forgiveness. The defence of inner conviction and integrity is disallowed, people have to weep and grovel, while silence is even more reprehensible than straight denial.

Yet the right to keep silent is the last resource of the innocent before despicable judges: when honest argument is useless, silence shows the moral distance between the innocent man and the executioner, setting the fury of the prosecutors against the serenity of the victim, and so preserving the possibility of future justification against the ephemeral triumph of imposture. False justice becomes exasperated when it breaks against the rock-like silence of the innocent, and thereby betrays its purposes and stands unmasked for all to see.

Where confession is deemed essential, the process of debasement is most clearly to be seen. No doubt all human justice involves a certain amount of debasement of the guilty man who confesses, since such confession is not made entirely freely, and does not represent spontaneous conversion from wrong-doing. Nor does it know how to receive such a confession. It cannot entirely forgive, and the less savoury aspects of the confessional act itself are repeated when justice rejects its plea for absolution and refuses the immediate act of forgiveness which might help the guilty person to find his own salvation. Confession is taken as the final proof of guilt, not as the first sign of the desire to make restitution. It seizes on the confession to put a good face on its severity, and does not use it as an act of repentance and a call for help. So justice, by a sad contradiction, punishes with greater severity at the very moment when free confession shows guilt to be less than it was. The evil counsel, 'Never own up', is justified by its results, not only by sordid calculation, and because justice is always a little hesitant before a hardened denier. Besides, there is a remnant of dignity in denying one's guilt, when one thinks of the use to which one's confession will be put. Thus, by rejecting confession as a burden it cannot carry, justice pushes the victim back towards the abyss. This may be necessary in defence of society, but the fact remains that this atrocious misunderstanding, this sombre dialogue between two deaf people, the accused and his judge, exemplifies the drama of human justice which is incapable of punishing without also debasing.

Ordinary justice such as this might perhaps argue that it sacrifices the guilty to indisputable moral values, and that admission of guilt implies acceptance also of the constraint imposed by these values, the punishment meted out to those who transgress them. But justices of political extermination have the peculiarity that they use the admissions of the accused as articles of propaganda. Physical elimination alone is insufficient, it has to be coupled with moral elimination, so that the ideas of the accused have also to be killed. The last words of the corpse, they have promised themselves, have to justify the executioners, not so much in pronouncing sentence as in showing adoration of the System. The victim must prove that he has come round to the ideology which kills him, and that he has therefore agreed to his own crucifixion. That is why confession without apostasy is not enough. The accused, after admitting his crime, has also to show himself clear of past delusions, and, seeing the light, asks for punishment and blesses the judges who have saved him. Further, by a refinement of cruelty, and for propaganda purposes, he is expected to state publicly that his confession is entirely voluntary and that he has not been badly treated! So the System wins all round; it kills; it is also the Truth; the machine which destroys is right.

It is clear that when confession is degraded into denial of previous faith so that it may be used for propaganda, simple torture is not enough, for this would leave a point of uncertainty: the victim might retract, refuse to sign the certificate required of him, or show that he was acting under duress. So this too has to be dealt with. To make apostasy durable, to give it the semblance of free action, a real transformation of personality is needed: freewill and conscience must vanish, another will and another conscience have to be infused into the living corpse whose soul has been destroyed. The justice which tortured was nothing to what we have to-day: the justice which dements.

We can only guess at the psychological technique of this nightmare, but our ignorance is no reason for taking on an air of superior scepticism and for telling those who are anxious about such things not to be childish. When two hypotheses are before one, one accepts the more likely. It is much harder to believe in these unexpected and stereotyped confessions than to believe that there are means adapted to plucking out and destroying the individual will. And if we do not know what rôle drugs play in them, or what drugs these may be, that gives us no cause for reassurance about those we already know and dread, for though they go much less far, they nevertheless belong to the same category.

5. RENEGADE AND MARTYR

I am not going to speak in praise of torture, but one must have lost all sense of what are unequalled and unassailable spiritual values not to realize that there is worse than torture in all this. The latter admittedly degrades when it destroys freedom of will, but it does not always degrade. We see this in the case of martyrs, since it leaves them a last and finest resource, which lifts them above the merely human level and places them where heroism and holiness clasp hands. We are here concerned with methods which cancel out even that last resource of the spirit, degrading people for good. One can foresee the Nero of the future using, not hot irons and wild beasts, but skilful techniques to produce spiritual apostasy. The dark hour would then be upon us when the Church *could* have no martyrs.

The problem of Christian martyrdom lies at the back of the survival of our civilization. Doubtless martyrdom belongs primarily to the realm of the supernatural and is a witness to Christ, but it can also be the last rampart of human values, when it stands as a protest in favour of a free spirit and against tyranny and barbarism. At no time in the history of the Church has there not been bloody testimony of faith somewhere in the world, and it is equally certain that the problem will arise before long in a different guise. The present situation of Christianity in a decadent civilization will force us at some moment to gather together once more our scattered ultimate values, hence it calls with tragic insistence and foresight for a profound revival of our ideas on Christian martyrdom. For it is quite evident that everything will be done to try and prevent the martyr from standing out as a shining example, and that the torturers will do their utmost to deprive him of his power of irradiation.

We have seen already how political disfranchisement has induced the public to see the martyr as a degraded creature, and how, by various accusations, it can make him seem a rogue or a criminal. This is no new idea: in the second century it was said that the Christians ate children. In the twentieth they are accused of sexual perversion or of trafficking in currency. More insidious still is the flexible and indefinite term 'traitor'. These things allow of religious persecution on grounds of public safety—again no new thing, since there has scarcely been any religious persecution in historical times which did not depend on direct or indirect political accusations. What is frightening to-day is the threat to Christian solidarity itself on the question of the exact meaning of the term religious persecution. It is well known that there are some who are prepared to excuse, if not to approve, religious purging on the ground of 'collaborationism', or of 'reaction' and 'feudalism'. Some Christians had not a good word to say for Monseigneur Stepinaç and found good reasons to explain the Mindszenty trial. Yet they are much concerned with the political trials of Rajk and Kostov, where the executioners themselves become the victims. Better late than never—but it is all the same very late. We shall doubtless, before long, see Christians, blinded or made fanatical by politics, applauding if not helping in the persecution of their own brothers. It is enough to make one tremble.

We can also forecast that the persecutors, knowing the powers and dangers of propaganda, will see to it that martyrdom is not publicized, so that it cannot become a contagious example. Martyrs will be made in secret, and the noisy trials of to-day will be thought of as pieces of clumsiness in making martyrs and then exhibiting them to the whole world. There is already a difference between the treatment of Cardinal Mindszenty by the Hungarian Government and that of Monseigneur Beran in Czechoslovakia. The Nazi method will come into favour, that is, suppression by clandestine kidnapping. Should the censors ever allow the news to leak out, all that the Christian community will know is that one of their fellows has vanished. It may guess that he has been persecuted, but will not know whether he has received the crown of death or whether he is still rotting in a pit.

The method of choice, of course, in all these affairs will be to force a repudiation of faith. So far we appear to be only at a stage where indirect denial is demanded, and all that has been asked openly is for political repentance, and religious matters have only been lightly touched on by making the accused testify to the freedom of religion in his country. It is pushing matters to the utmost to force the victims to make a statement for propaganda purposes which camouflages the real anti-religious nature of the operation.

A little more and the accused may be made to blaspheme and to perform sacrilege in the same way as the early Christians were made to bow down before idols. In any case, the pattern of future prosecutions is already fixed, and that is, by a terrifying use of lying: executioners have the power, in order to give credit to their own lies, to compel their victims to lie in harmony with them.

By an extraordinary paradox, martyrdom, which has hitherto been a matter of heroic resistance to false beliefs, will now become linked with what appears to be the most shameful forms of compromise and compounding with crime. The martyr was one who was a witness to truth: he is now to be forced to appear as a renegade.

This sort of ruination is disturbing to the Christian conscience, but refusal to become resigned to it is in itself a heroic protest in the moment of defeat. We have evidence of this in Cardinal Mindszenty's declaration before his arrest, when, foreseeing what his executioners might do to him, he denied in advance his possible repudiation of his faith.[1] This surely is the ultimate act of heroism, to be ready to confront torture when all hope of heroic action is lost. A Protestant theological writer has even gone so far as to think that there may be times when suicide may be the supreme form of Christian testimony,[2] the only means

---

1. '*Half an hour before he was arrested, the Cardinal had time to write the following on the back of a used envelope which he was able to conceal from the police searchers:* '(1) I have been concerned in no plot. (2) I will never give up my function. (3) I refuse to make any statement. (4) Should it ever be said that I have acknowledged the facts or resigned my function and even if my own signature were given as proof, this must be looked on as a sign of human frailty, and I declare now that any confession I may make is null and void.' *White Book: Documents published at the Request of Cardinal Mindszenty*, p. 182 (Amiot-Dumont, Paris, 1949).

2. '*Shall we end by reaching the supreme absurdity in which we shall see suicide as a valid witness for Christianity because it will be the only way of preventing a corpse from betraying that which dwelled in it?*' Pastor Bosc, in *Réforme*, 12 March, 1949, referring to the trial of the Pastors in Sofia.

by which the soul can still stand firm before a living corpse is made to speak in its stead: the last effort of the hero at the place where heroism itself dies.

This is the point where explanations and resolutions made by man are vain, and only the mystery of Grace remains. We have no proper idea of what this power may achieve even in a being disintegrated to the point where he is no longer human. The ways of the Spirit are not to be foreseen. Until now they seemed to follow the path of heroism; but now, by an apparent turning away from grace, weakness may still be its own witness.

The whole problem can only be resolved by a complete change of perspective. Instead of considering the testimony of the witness himself, we shall have to think in terms of how that testimony is received by the community to which it is given. When one is faced by the strange witnessing of one who denies, the thing which matters is to preserve his rôle as martyr and, despite all its equivocal nature and its disguises, to cherish its power to illumine. The testimony must be accepted even when the witness can no longer testify. To the community which wishes to retain its insight and coherence, this new kind of martyrdom must have exemplary significance. Understood and suffered as such, no form of persecution of faith, however clever an impostor the persecutor may be, however lamentable the denials of the victim, the fundamental meaning and the basic power of bringing about communion with God remain unshaken. The problem to-day is not whether there will always be unshakable martyrs for Christianity but whether Christians will remain unshakable in their recognition of their martyrs.

6. TRUTH SERUM, INDEED!

From one angle, this story of drugs is a summary of our whole civilization. The need for artificial heavens into which one can escape is no new thing, but hitherto it seemed to be reserved, under aesthetic forms, to artists anxious to replenish the vials of their sensibility. Under the common garb of the vice of drunkenness it is marked for censure, since it degrades, but now, under the seal of medicine, the gate is open to anybody who comes along. I know people who think they will find mental health by undergoing 'cures' by narco-analysis: thus practising a form of drug addiction under medical direction. Any young fool, anxious about his examinations, can, even without a proper prescription, and for a few shillings, buy at the chemists a little memory and an increase of spirit. That is because in a society where everything is aimed at 'taking one out of oneself', drugs have a fine field. Everybody hopes, by using them, to recapture some rag of his scattered personality, some fictitious means of peace, some kind of euphoria either through self-surrender or self-excitation—a drugging of the constant fret of the man who finds himself always at odds with life, with no standards of normality, absorbed into the herd. Drugs provide an artificial compensation for the loss of spiritual realities which is the mark of contemporary civilization.

The worst of the drama is that by a curious paradox the very drugs which are used in this desperate attempt to catch hold of oneself can also serve the worst enterprises of self-abandonment. Pentothal, maxiton, benzedrine, offer the repressed and the depressed a transitory sense of well-being, of balance, of new enthusiasm; but they also offer the tyrant the means to disintegrate all that might resist absorption, all that remains of self-possession, self-affirmation. Escaping from the herd by drugging, and pushed back to the herd by the same means, man is caught on the infernal wheel of the social Moloch determined to hold on to his prey. He tries to escape into an unreal heaven only to fall back into a very real hell.

The paradox of the psycho-dynamic drug not only shows the drama of modern man, it also shows a bottle-neck in our perception of things. We said above that the investigation of the mind by dislocating the will is an attempt to penetrate into the depths of the soul directly, and not by the mediation of signs and symbols. Such a remark brings up a strange analogy—which doubtless the reader will have seen —between the techniques of physics for breaking up matter and the psychological technique for breaking up the soul. There is more in this than a rough, if spectacular resemblance, and the real origin of both the destruction of the material particle and the psychic entity lies in a similar bent in research. The same movement of consciousness urges the mind to try and enter the sanctuary of the real by penetrating beyond the signs by which it manifests: beyond the data of the senses to understand matter, beyond the signs of behaviour, to know consciousness. The strange thing is that in both cases the urge to go beyond the outer manifestations ends in the flight of the reality which is being pursued, or else in so changing that reality that it is as if it had been actually destroyed. As a result, the knowledge obtained is less definite, less real than that which could have been reached by a proper interpretation of simple external signs. Matter, to-day, can only be explained in terms of mathematical probability: that is, without certainty. The state of the soul, scattered by dissociation of the personality, loses all semblance to the mental unity which alone can give the various parts significance. How then can one say that one has reached reality? I find it difficult to believe that the equations of wave-mechanics represent a world more real than that of a ray of light or the song of a bird; or that the dismemberment of an intoxicated mind gives me a picture of the soul more real than that of its controlled expressions.

There is a devilish quality about a science which can only reach the real by destroying it. Doubtless the thing is congenital to the human spirit, and latent in its history. It would be childish to want to put the clock back on the way science has developed, but one should at least avoid the illusion that the objects on which it seizes or the quality of the knowledge it provides are authentic.

BACKGROUND

This reflects into the scope of techniques which science produces. To be sure, we may see the atom bomb as an apocalyptic punishment on a humanity which has violated forbidden mysteries, but this will not protect us. In the same way, philosophic argument alone will not prevent barbarism triumphant from using pharmacological research in its techniques of police extortion. The threat of cosmic destruction and spiritual death arise primarily from a certain state of civilization. Our own is so precarious that this is strong reason for not frivolously introducing certain methods into a world which would use them for evil purposes. Yet alongside this external reason there lies the philosophical principle which forbids the use of chemically induced mental analysis in judicial technique. That is, that they do not lead to *realities*, or that if they do, they automatically destroy or distort them. Psychiatrists may be sufficiently fore-armed against this distortion by the caution with which they practise their art and the subtlety of their psycho-analytical interpretations: that is their affair. But under the special conditions of judicial *expertise* (haste, poor equipment, difficulty in repeating the examination and hence of correcting mistakes), and where the conclusions drawn from the analysis, whether by the doctor or the judge, may have grave repercussions not to be foreseen, things are otherwise. Moreover, the method may be used by incompetent or dishonest people. All these things risk to disfigure truth and may lead to some of the worst psychological and hence judicial errors.

Such are the basic metaphysical criteria on which to judge the *truth* given by the use of drugs which bring about mental dissociation. The meaning of the phrase *truth serum* becomes clear in all its absurdity. One might as well call the atom bomb the detector of reality!

Everybody will agree that with this kind of truth we are travelling towards a world which is both strange and disturbing. When consciousness is dismembered and out of the control of the self, its intimacies lying open to the eyes of everybody, everything must be at once both false and true. Nothing is concealed, but nothing is in its proper place. The light which abolishes all shadow also abolishes all outline. Everything is known, none of it makes sense: it has the transparency of a phantasm. The icy clarity which removes all mystery thereby destroys all reality. Forced consciousness is falsified consciousness. The kind of reality which rules in hell must be of this order.

Appendix

NARCOANALYSIS[1]

By Edward V. Saher

I. IMPORTANCE OF NARCOANALYSIS

NARCOANALYSIS is a topic which requires careful consideration by the legal profession. Its present importance has generally been overestimated by the public at large, which speaks of the truth serum as if it were sufficient to inject a person with certain drugs in order to make him confess. This is not the case. A drug which has such an effect has not yet been found.

In order to arrive at a proper evaluation of narcoanalysis from the standpoint of the law, the Executive Council of the International Bar Association has directed me to consult with members of the medical profession.

II. STANDPOINT OF THE MEDICAL PROFESSION

The best method is to let the members of this profession speak for themselves.

Martin J. Gerson, M.D., of New York and Victor M. Victoroff, M.D. of Cleveland, have published a highly interesting article 'Experimental Investigation into the Validity of Confessions Obtained under Sodium Amytal Narcosis' reprinted from the *Journal of Clinical Psychopathology*, Vol. 9, No. 3. July 1948. I have quoted parts of their article, and summarized other parts.

In my opinion the legal profession should be grateful to these two outstanding medical experts for writing an article which gives in plain and easily understandable language a survey of the medical side of the problem, but who also understand that this problem cannot be solved by one of these professions alone, but only by the co-operation of

1. Paper presented at the Third International Conference of the International Bar Association in London, in July 1950. Published with the kind permission of the author.

both. They have also given proof of a remarkable understanding of the legal aspects of the question.

In the course of psychiatric study of patients hospitalized on the Neuropsychiatric Service of Tilton General Hospital, Fort Dix, N.J., the authors have uncovered the following data:

> After it became apparent that we were uncovering data which could be considered inimical to the interests of the patient if it fell into the hands of the police or military authorities, we made an effort to investigate the possibilities and limitations of the use of narcoanalysis as an instrument of interrogation.
>
> None of the material developed in these interviews was used in the prosecution of the charges against the patients, since it was considered by us to be a breach of medical ethics, and because this material, derived without the full knowledge and consent of the patient could not have been presented in court without violating the Twenty-Fourth Article of War and the Bill of Rights of the Constitution of the United States.

I quote from this article:

Technics and Observations

Prior to actual induction of the medication, the patients were interviewed by the psychiatrist. The patient-doctor relationship was maintained and the fact that the patient was in most instances a prisoner, or under police scrutiny, was quietly accepted but not stressed. It was established at the outset that everything the doctor learned was confidential, and could not be revealed without the explicit permission of the soldier. He was urged to describe his social and family background, army career and to discuss his version of the charges pending against him.

It was pointed out to the soldier that the circumstances leading to his arrest had been described to the doctor, and casual reference was made to obvious discrepancies in the explanation vouchsafed by the patient and the evidence collected by the police. Evasions, rationalizations or simple refusal to explain the contradictions were pursued only briefly by the medical officer. The doctor suggested without emphasis that it might be wiser for the patient to co-operate in the investigation, that this course was the more soldierly, honourable one to follow; that it would only complicate the work of the court martial to validate their charges; and that a policy of negativism would be likely to prejudice his case and increase his punishment if he were found guilty. The physician then proceeded to other topics.

The history of neuropathic traits, habits and symptoms was gone into frankly, as were psychosomatic problems. Much of the suspicion against the medical officer was lessened when his interest in the patient's 'nervousness', 'irritability', 'tendency to get into trouble', and 'bad breaks' was expressed and an investigation of medical problems pursued.

An uncovering approach to the patient's psychic ailments was attempted, and psychotherapy offered. Concurrent with the interviews with the psychiatrist, a social history was taken by a trained psychiatric case worker, in nearly ever case, who detailed information given by the patient.

The patients were not informed that narcoanalysis would be performed until a few minutes before that procedure was undertaken. It was explained to them that the drug would make them feel sleepy, and encourage them to discuss things with the doctor that might enable him to gain fuller understanding of their personalities and motivations.

Patients who had claimed to suffer amnesia were told that the drug would help restore their memory for the forgotten episodes. The doctor was positive, forthright but considerate. He indicated by his manner that the patient had no choice but to submit to the procedure and was expected to co-operate when told to take off his shirt or jacket and lie on the bed. The attitude of the patients varied from unquestioning compliance to downright refusal to submit to the drug.

Six patients obeyed without temporizing and accepted the doctor's explanation; three were suspicious and wary but offered no protests; three indicated they thought the procedure unnecessary and asked to be excused; four were hostile and spoke bitterly about the proceedings, objecting to being given 'truth serum', demanding their rights to 'see the Inspector General', or becoming abusive; one patient flatly refused to have 'needles stuck in me', and talked antagonistically, hinting against the procedure, but sullenly submitted when he demanded (and was given) a 'direct order' to comply.

Sodium amytal was the narcotic agent used in every case. One gram (1.0 Gm) of the drug in 10 cc. of distilled water was available, and was injected slowly into the antecubital vein. It was found necessary to bring the patient through the stages of light sleepiness; mild disorientation with a tendency toward euphoria; confusion and somnolence, with irritability if roused by painful stimuli (rubbing the sternum or pinching the skin); to complete narcosis (second plane of the third stage anaesthesia). The patient was then permitted to sleep. As he became semiconscious, and could be stimulated to speak he was held in this stage by discreet additional use of the drug while questioning proceeded.

The subject matter introduced by the psychiatrist in the early stages was relatively innocuous and referred to material in the soldier's background which had previously been discussed with him and had bearing on his basic personality structure. Early childhood incidents of traumatic character, relationships with siblings, attitude toward parents and others, father and mother surrogates in the patient's constellation of adult influence, relevant sexual experience, friendships with other soldiers, incidents in his army history, and attitude toward the army career and environment all provided leads for questioning. Whenever possible the soldier himself was manipulated into bringing up the charges pending against him and it was not until he had that the questioning was directed to that sphere. It was found to be more successful to ask the patient to 'talk about that later', and interpose a topic which would diminish suspicion, delaying interrogation of his criminal activity until he was in the proper stage of narcosis.

Speech was thick, mumbling, disconnected and characterized by echolalia and paralogia when going from unconsciousness back to consciousness. But discretion was markedly lessened and if the patient did answer questions at this time, the answers were usually revealing.

This most valuable interrogation period lasted only five to ten minutes, after which unless more amytal were injected and the patient put to sleep again, he rapidly revived, became aware that he had been questioned about his secrets, and, depending upon his underlying personality structure, his fear of discovery, or his degree of disillusion in the doctor, became negativistic, hostile or physically aggressive.

Some patients had to be forcibly restrained during this period to prevent them from injuring themselves or others. The doctor continued questioning and sometimes, because of the patient's fierce, regressive, diffuse anger, the assumption that he had already been 'tricked' into confession, and his still limited sense of discretion, he defiantly acknowledged his guilt and challenged the observer to 'do something about it'. As the excitement stage passed, the patient either fell back on his original story or verified the confessed material.

Approximately half the patients were given 500 mg. of caffeine with sodium benzoate intramuscularly in order to hasten recovery from the narcotic effects of the drug. This practice was abandoned after it was found that the patient became garrulous, euphoric and hyperactive, staggering ataxically around the ward several hours. Without the stimulant, he was encouraged to go to bed and sleep, after which, though mentally dull, he was fairly well oriented. On the day following narcoanalysis, another interview was held with the patient, the material unearthed was discussed *in toto* and the possible psychic etiology of his criminal behaviour was taken up.

Two major differences from ordinary narcoanalysis in the method described above must be stressed. First, the period of obliviscence of consciousness was invariably longer than average. Second, the patient was maintained in the period of beginning recovery from the nadir of narcotic sleep. This was a period which proved richest in productivity of the material most threatening to him. It is seldom necessary to narcotize a patient for so long or as deeply in simple narcoanalysis.

The technique of questioning varied in each case according to what was known about the patient through history and interview, the seriousness of legal charges, the patient's attitude under narcoanalysis and his rapport with the doctor. Sometimes it was useful to assume that the patient had already confessed in the amnestic period of the analysis, and while his memory and sense of self-protection were still limited, he was urged to continue to elaborate details he had 'already described'. Key questions were reworded when it was obvious that the patient was withholding the truth, and the fact of a given denial was quickly passed over and ignored.

In our series of patients, nine admitted the validity of their confessions, eight repudiated the confessions and persisted in their original stories when confronted with the evidence confessed during the narcotic period.

The following factors operated in greater or lesser degree in the cases to interfere with the completeness and authenticity of confessions:

1. Inept questioning.
2. Tendency of patient to persevere on unrelated topics.
3. Echolalia and paralogia.
4. Mumbled, thick, inaudible speech.
5. Fantasies.
6. Contradictory but apparently truthful evidence.
7. Poor rapport between doctor and patient.

The modification of consciousness by a narcotic is characterized by confusion, bewilderment, inability to assay and select thought, impoverishment of vocabulary, automatic rather than reasoned responses, disturbed memory, expanded or contracted (distorted) sequence of chronology, and the loss of discrimination between what is real and what is illusory. Several patients revealed fantasies, fears and delusions sometimes approaching th quality of delirium, much of which could readily be distinguished from reality by its fantastic quality. At times, however, it was necessary to check the facts by reference to objective sources for information because otherwise there was no way for the examiner to distinguish the truth from the fantasy.

It must be admitted that had investigation not previously established as fact that J. L.'s parents were his own and that the child he claimed did not exist; that E. F.'s wife was not actually in prison, and his child was as yet unborn; and that G. H.'s stepfather of whom he said, 'I'll kill the bastard when I see him on the street', had been dead a year, the examiner would have been unable to determine that these experiences were fantasied, and might well have accepted them verbatim.

Testimony concerning dates and specific places are untrustworthy and often contradictory because of the patient's loss of time-sense. Names and events are of questionable veracity. Contradictory statements are often made without the patient actually trying to conceal the truth, but succeeding in this by his confusion between what has actually happened, and what he thinks or fears may have happened.

This is borne out, for example, by P. V.'s conflicting description under narcosis, of his part in the robbery of the Post Exchange. He vehemently denied having been present at the actual scene of the robbery, but later, during the same session, described plausible details of 'what happened' the night the Post Exchange was robbed. Investigation by the Criminal Investigation Division had independently established that the soldier had not been a direct accomplice, but had bought goods from the men who committed the robbery. His description of the details of the crime was a reconstruction of second-hand information and pure fantasy.

In this instance, if the auditor chose to give credence to his 'admission' of having participated in the crime, and if it were admissible as evidence in court without further verification, the man might have been prosecuted for a more serious crime than the one of which he was guilty (receiving stolen property).

Persistent, careful questioning can reduce the ambiguities, but cannot eliminate them.

In the final stages of narcoanalysis, it was necessary to reassure the soldier that his confession was not going to be released to the police, and that the problem was now one which the doctor would share and help him to decide. An attempt to assuage the guilty feelings that arose out of recollection of the offence was made by indicating that the confession may well have been an indication that the patient was ready to make amends, was remorseful and had 'learned his lesson'.

An attempt to develop insight and the self-evaluation of the patient's admission of his guilt was most successful in our neurotic patients and immature personalities, and least successful with the confirmed psychopaths.

Discussion of Mechanics and Psychodynamics of Confession

A number of explanations have been offered for the production of confession under narcotic drugs.

A masochistic wish to seek punishment which may motivate psychopathic behaviour puts the criminal in a peculiar dilemma. His natural caution urges him to seek seclusion and avoid all future connexion with the crime he may have committed, but his desire to claim credit for the act, plus a potent wish-for-punishment may cause him to neglect his safety and perform acts which may inevitably lead to his capture.

Aside from the desire to achieve self-aggrandizement and recognition and the wish-for-punishment, confessions may follow when fears attendant upon their declaration are reduced. Fears of retaliation, social stigma, pecuniary loss and punishment are better met by the reinforced ego which may make a realistic compromise with the community, balancing the precarious safety of the secret against the squaring of accounts with the social environment.

Kubie, Grinker, Freed and Barbara have commented on this phenomenon, suggesting that narcosis promotes removal of tension, anxiety, and defence barriers and helps the reintegration of the ego functions.

Kubie suggests that 'Cortex and diencephalon are depressed by the drugs, loosening the patient's grip on reality, making it possible for the individual to release those anxiety-laden impulses and attitudes which would be of unbearable nature if expressed in the conscious state'.

Grinker states that the anxiety appreciated by the cortex arising from the diencephalon is markedly reduced and the discriminatory part of the ego which represents cortical functioning is thus inhibited. This could readily be applied to the mechanics of confession if the physiologic basis were sound.

In support, Freed proposes that the release of strong affect demonstrates the specific effect of barbiturates on the diencephalon. In our cases the affective responses could not be correlated with the depth of narcosis, the amount of resistance or the productivity of the patient in confession. However, strong affect was brought out against the physician as an expression of hostility and by fear of imminent betrayal. Rage reactions were common and intense after confession or as an immediate precursor to confession.

It was suggested by House that the patient under scopolamine, '. . . cannot create a lie and that there is no power to think or reason'.

We must indicate that our experience with amytal does not bear out his statement in that our patients could sometimes lie and that their reasoning powers were sometimes present though much distorted.

Patients who have a strong desire to confess, but who for either emotional or politic reasons cannot bring themselves to it may even on a conscious level welcome narcosis as an excuse to inform. Into this category fell men who feared to violate the 'criminal's code' against squealers even when it was to their interest to do so.

Other patients, who had placed themselves in difficult situations by malingering amnesia, used the analytic sessions as a device to 'recover' their memory without loss of 'face'.

On page 372 Dr. Gerson and Dr. Victoroff mention the medical application of narcosis as a deception indicator whose possibilities have been relatively unexplored or unreported in literature. This fact is of interest for the present paper only insofar as it demonstrates that many problems in connexion with narcoanalysis have not yet been fully investigated. The authors finally summarize their opinion as follows:

> Although amytal narcoanalysis has been successful for the revelation of deception, validity of information garnered by this method is not so decisive that it should be admissible in court without further investigation and substantiation. The doctor cannot tell when the patient's recollections turn into fantasy, cannot positively state whether he is stimulating deep narcosis and actually maintaining his lies, and cannot, without social investigation, determine which of contrary stories told under narcoanalysis are true.
>
> This complicates the position of the doctor who hears during analysis testimony or information from the patient which might indicate that he had been guilty of crime. To expose his patient to police investigation might even with the best of intentions on the part of the physician lead to humiliation and embarrassment of the patient, and possibly a lawsuit for malpractice against the doctor.
>
> It would seem at the present writing that there is no such thing as a 'truth serum'. Certainly, more study of amytal narcoanalysis as a method for interrogation should be done before its findings can be offered to the courts as valid, unquestioned evidence.
>
> There is quite a tradition and precedent which might make submission to narcoanalysis mandatory some day in the routine investigation of certain crimes. The taking of fingerprints; premarital Wassermann examinations; the reporting of venereal disease contact to the Board of Health; blood, urine or breath analysis of suspected alcoholics; the enforced hospitalization of active tubercular and typhoid fever patients; and the submission to examination by alienists and psychologists are all limitations of freedom, and in a sense force the individual to give evidence about himself whether he wants to or not.
>
> Much discussion will have to be invested by psychiatrists and lawyers to determine when narcoanalysis per-

formed in the interest of the state violates the fundamental rights of the patient and the ethics of the doctor.

There are also a few other statements which may be mentioned.

In their 'Narco-investigation et expertise psychiatrique' (*Rev. Sc. Crim. Dr. Pen. Comp.*, Paris, 1948, p. 131) M. Bouvet and F. Gravejal give a survey of a number of cases from which a negative result was obtained, although the patients had asked for the treatment.

A well-known member of the medical profession in the United Kingdom, Dr. Denis Carroll, reported the following interesting case:

During the war he treated an officer who suffered from mental disturbances and suggested to him that he should undergo narcoanalytical treatment. The patient said that he did not feel that he could submit himself to such treatment as he was the bearer of important military secrets. The matter was submitted to the commanding officer, who authorized the treatment and who also authorized the doctor, during the treatment, to ask questions about the secrets which were not known to the doctor. The treatment as such developed satisfactorily, but the doctor could not elicit any information from his patient concerning the secrets.

During World War II Grinker, Spiegel and others of the American Air Force, and Wilde, Sargent, Slater and many others of the British Armed Forces developed this method on a large scale in an effort to improve and expedite the treatment of psychiatric casualties (Carl P. Adatto, M.D., 'Narcoanalysis as a Diagnostic Aid in Criminal Cases', *Journal of Clinical Pathology*, April 1947).

To-day the seasoned opinion holds that the therapeutic significance of narcoanalysis is limited.

The well-known psychiatrist and author, Professor Franz Alexander, Director of the Psychoanalytic Institute of Chicago, Illinois, has gained the impression 'that whenever a person suspected of an illegal act really wants to withhold information the use of narcotics cannot overcome his resistance, and that, on the other hand, more reliable information can be obtained by prolonged psychiatric interviews conducted in the waking state'.

Dr. Roy R. Frinker, Chairman of Division of Neuropsychiatry, Michael Reese Hospital, Chicago, Ill., made the following statement:

> Under narcoanalysis, the truth is not invariably brought forth. The subject may be able to disguise the truth for a considerable length of time and perhaps always. I cannot say that any particular area may be falsified. I would agree that narcoanalysis from a medical standpoint should be used only to report on the condition of the patient until such time as society has an adequate attitude toward a suspect murderer. In regard to the circumstances which may prevent discovery of the truth, I believe that no general statements can be made. The subjects with highly developed guilt feelings will of course spill easily.

I quote further from his letter of 14 September 1949: 'The capability and experience of the medical expert are of course a great significance in determining the efficacy of the treatment . . . a subject may be hypnotized under the drug'.

I submitted some questions to Dr. Grinker, and give below the question and answer:

Q. What should be submitted to a court as a result of the treatment?

A. A summary is probably all that is necessary rather than a complete statement although it is possible for a complete transcript to be made. I think the results should be submitted by transcript and testimony. In general, I might say that there has not been enough work on suspect criminals to validate any of my impressions. I have had a few in the Army and have fortunately been able to disclose circumstances which mitigated the crimes.

Q. May witnesses be present during the treatment?

A. Witnesses can be present and they may be lay people, except for the problem of medical ethics which should be modified if such a procedure were used for legal purposes.

Q. Is it possible to have a cross-narcoanalysis?
A. It is possible to have a cross-narcoanalysis by another medical expert and I believe the subject's own legal adviser and own medical examiner should be present.
Q. Can narcoanalysis show harmful results to the patient, and can a patient be influenced with regard to the attitude taken after treatment?
A. Narcoanalysis has never been shown to be harmful. Yes, a defendant can be influenced with regard to the attitude taken after a treatment, as in hypnosis. Under our present legal system, a subject must give his free consent. In my mind, it may be advantageous for the court to be privileged to request such an analysis as they may request a lie detector test for suspects, but again this is dependent upon society's attitude toward a suspect criminal.

I also cite from *Psychological Abstracts* (Vol. 23, 1949 No. 2792):

Schneider, Pierre B. (U. Basel, Switzerland), Psychiatrie legale et narcoanalyse. (Legal psychiatry and narcoanalysis), *Schweiz. Arch. Neurol. Psychiat.*, 1948, 62, 352-371:

Examination under subnarcosis (pentothal induced) was made on four criminals or individuals presumed such and on five non-delinquent subjects to ascertain whether so-called 'truth-serum' can actually elicit the truth in the sense of a confession and whether subjects are rendered more suggestible in the subnarcotic state to the examiner. The results somewhat differing from subject to subject led the author to the conviction that narcoanalysis could be useful for examination of delinquents reticent or refusing to confess; that a subject under pentothal does not admit a crime he has not committed; that confession pure and simple is not the rule; that the subject will most often sketch a confession, only to recover himself immediately; that his affective reactions, a word-too-much, an unfortunate gesture will betray him. It is not therefore a question of confessions in the strict juridical sense of the term but of psychological indices which, if they are reproduced in an expert psychiatric report, will represent a serious charge against the subject. Finally, it appears possible that a criminal is able, in spite of narcoanalysis, not to make confession and never to allow himself to be caught in a trap.— F. C. Sumner.

In order to avoid misunderstanding it must be pointed out that narcoanalysis has been extensively applied in the U.S.A. for therapeutic purposes but it has been applied *only in a very limited number of criminal cases* and only if the defendant has given his consent.

Summary of the Standpoint of the Medical Profession

The standpoint of the medical profession can be summarized as follows:

Narcoanalysis is not a sure method of bringing out 'the truth and nothing but the truth'. Any confession made is not necessarily true; and if no confession is made this does not necessarily prove that the patient has not committed the crime with which he may be charged. Does this mean that narcoanalysis has no importance at all from the angle of the administration of justice?

The answer to this question is again in the negative, because in many cases the confession is true, and often facts are brought out which are very helpful to the public prosecutor in proving his case. It seems fair to say that in the present stage of development narcoanalysis can be of great help in finding the truth.

But it is also a dangerous means of investigation as the right interpretation of statements made depends largely on the skill of the analyst.

It is therefore a means of investigation which should not be applied without certain specific guarantees, if, indeed, it is applied at all.

III. ATTITUDE OF MEDICAL AND LEGAL ORGANIZATIONS TOWARD NARCOANALYSIS

Many organizations have voted resolutions against the use of narcoanalysis. In a very interesting article in the

Rechtskundig Weekblad of Antwerp, Belgium, Judge Versele of Leuven, Belgium, has listed a number of such resolutions; among others that of the French Association for Forensic Medicine (*Annales de Médecine Légale de France*, 1945, No. 44, p. 44).

On 22 March 1949, the Academy of Medicine in Paris unanimously adopted a resolution against the application of narcoanalysis in criminal proceedings. It rejected by a large majority, a resolution to the effect that narcoanalysis could be used in order to facilitate medical diagnosis at the request of the defendant and his lawyer. (*Rev. Dr. pen.*, 1948–1949, p. 880.)

In his 'Le dépistage scientifique du mensonge, ou la question moderne' (*Rev. Crim. Pol. tech.*, Genève, 1948, p. 163) Justice Jan Graven of Geneva also cautioned the profession against the indiscriminate use of narcoanalysis.

After having heard an address by Maître de Coulhac-Mazerieux (published in the *Gaz. Pal.*, Paris 21/23 Juli 1948) the Paris Bar, on 6 July 1948, voted against the application of narcoanalysis, which it considered as 'une atteinte au principe de l'inviolabilité de la personne humaine' (*Rev. Intern. Dr. pen.*, Paris, 1948, p. 431).

On 18 July 1949, the Belgian Association for Penal Law accepted a motion made by our learned friend, Professor S. Sasserath, against the application of drugs.

On the other hand my co-rapporteur, Dr. Christo P. Yotis of Athens, Greece, in his paper presented to the Conference, writes on the assumption that narcoanalysis may be given general application.

Judge Versele of Leuven, Belgium, takes an optimistic look on the development of criminal proceedings. He sees the judge of the future as a friend of the defendant, who tenders him his help. Within the framework of this development narcoanalysis should not be an instrument in the hands of a prosecutor, but would be used in a spirit of confidence with full respect for human dignity which is now so often endangered.

IV. CONSTRUCTIVE SOLUTION: APPLICATION OF NARCOANALYSIS WITH CAREFULLY DRAFTED LIMITATIONS

Although the weight of authority to-day is against the application of narcoanalysis as a means of eliciting confessions, extensive development of narcoanalysis in the U.S.A. as a therapeutic measure makes it appear very probable that it will find a place in the scope of criminal proceedings. The legal profession should look ahead and now give its constructive advice.

It is suggested that this should be to the effect that narcoanalysis be permitted with carefully drafted limitations.

A. *Rule against self-incrimination*

Article V of the Bill of Rights of the U.S.A. says . . . 'No person . . . shall be compelled in any criminal case to be a witness against himself.'

In the above-mentioned article in *Rechtskundig Weekblad* Judge Versele gives a summary of the national rules that a defendant is not under obligation to do anything which he does not wish to do. This rule implies that narcoanalysis can only be applied to a defendant if he has given his consent to it. It also implies that it cannot be applied to a minor, who cannot properly give his consent.

B. *Rules of Ethics of the Medical Profession*

The basic New York rule is laid down in Article 352 of the Civil Practice Act, which provides that physicians shall not disclose professional information. (See Lloyd Paul Stryker, *Courts and Doctors*, New York, 1932.) This Article applies:
(a) if a patient-doctor relationship exists. It has been held that no such relationship exists in a criminal case when a physician examines a prisoner at the request of the District Attorney for the purpose of testifying with regard to the question of the prisoner's sanity. So held People *v.* Sliney, 137 N.Y. 570; People *v.* Hock, 159 N.Y. 291, 302, 44 N/E. 976, Kelly *v.* Dykes, 174 App.

Div. 786, 161 N.Y. S.551. (See also Sidney Smith, *Forensic Medicine*, Boston 1939.)

(b) only to information necessary to enable the physican to prescribe for or treat his patient and not to any other information. Green *v.* Metropolitan Street Ry. Co., 171 N.Y. 201, 63 N.E. 958.

In this case the doctor was held competent to testify to what the injured person told him as to how the accident happened, on the ground that such information was 'unnecessary for any purpose of surgical treatment'.

Article 354 of the Civil Practice Act clearly states that the privilege is that of the patient and not of the physician. The doctor shall not testify, unless the patient waives his privilege.

It has however been held that the granting of the privilege was never intended to serve as a shield for murderers and other criminals. Pierson *v.* People 7A, N.Y. 424, People *v.* Harris 136 N.Y. 423. The plain purpose of the statute was held to be the prevention of any disclosure by the physician 'which would injure the feelings, damage the character or impair the standing of the patient while living or disgrace his memory when dead'.

In 1944 the Penal Law of the State of New York was amended as follows:

1. Every physician attending or treating a case of bullet wound, gunshot wound, powder burn, or any other injury arising from or caused by the discharge of a gun, pistol, or other firearm, or whenever such case is treated in a hospital, sanitarium or other institution, the manager, superintendent or other person in charge shall report such case at once to the police authorities of the city, town or village where such physician, hospital, sanitarium or institution is located.

2. Every physician attending or treating a case of a wound actually or apparently inflicted by a knife, icepick, or other sharp or pointed instrument, which wound or injury is likely to or which may result in death, or whenever such case is treated in a hospital, sanitarium or other

institution, the manager, superintendent, or other person in charge shall report such case at once to the police authorities of the city, town, or village where such physician, hospital, sanitarium or institution is located.

3. Failure to make such a report shall be a misdemeanour.

This is a clear exception to the rule stated above. The medical profession objected to the provisions of this amendment.

Drs. Gerson and Victoroff state:

> The psychiatrist and psychoanalyst are exposed to a serious dilemma, since an intrinsic part of their diagnostic and therapeutic procedure is to obtain from the patient a description of his actions and thoughts, especially those which have been traumatic and for which he may have guilt feelings. According to the 'letter of the law' the psychiatrist should be expected to hand his patients over for prosecution when they have spoken of long hidden assaults, thefts, embezzlements and deceptions.
>
> During narcoanalysis, quite by accident, as it were, the physician may discover evidence of some crime which his patient had no intention of disclosing. What criteria would have to be satisfied before the physician could in conscience say: My duty to respect the confidence this patient put in me, and my own allegiance to professional ideals are overweighed by the dire consequences of permitting him to go unpunished for his crime. The discovery by a physician that an innocent man had been punished for an offence committed by his patient might be a case in point.

C. *Narcoanalysis of Witnesses or third parties*

The question of narcoanalysis is generally discussed only in connexion with its application to the defendant. Drs. Gerson and Victoroff point out that during narcoanalysis a physician may discover evidence of some crime. Possibly he may discover that an innocent man had been indicted or punished for the crime. The question then arises: Should he inform the public prosecutor? and what about a narcoanalysis of witnesses, with or without their permission?

D. *Limitation of cases in which narcoanalysis should be permitted*

Drs. Gerson and Victoroff made the following suggestions:

1. *Where an individual is guilty of crime and believes he can conceal his guilt even if subjected to 'truth serum':—* His notice for submitting to the test might be to strengthen his defence in court. He might, by the terms of his agreement, be able to call the doctor who conducted the analysis as a defence witness, and bring up the transcript indicating his 'innocence' in open court. On the other hand, refusal to submit to narcoanalysis might be mentioned by the prosecution in an effort to undermine his defence and prejudice the jury against him. This tactic might be used in forcing the patient to submit in the hope that he could avoid incriminating himself. Ludwig's experience with malingerers, and ours, bears out the possibility that he might be successful in refraining from answering by a completely negativistic attitude. However, it is probable that he would only succeed in trapping himself if he tried to maintain an alibi with the assumption that he would be able to use his wits and reasoning powers to ward off incriminating questions while drugged.

2. *The suspect who is innocent:—*A man who has difficulty in establishing his innocence would make a strong mark in his own favour by submitting to lie detection or narcoanalysis. His attitude while under the influence of the drug would indicate whether his co-operation were simulated or real, entirely apart from the actual transcript and answers to questions.

3. *The suspect who has lost his memory for the event and cannot say whether he is innocent or guilty:—*An individual may become implicated in a criminal action while under the influence of drugs or liquor, or while suffering a genuine fugue state or amnestic attack. Under narcosis he might divulge facts which would indicate his unconscious retention of memories relative to the events in question, and these in turn could clear or incriminate him.

4. *The false avowers of guilt:—*These are the publicity-conscious exhibitionists, the neurotic, morbid-minded individuals, the pranksters, and the pre-psychotic indi-

viduals who always crop up after an infamous crime and must be weeded out by the police at considerable expense and with difficulty. Narcoanalysis might quickly determine not only their innocence but their basic motive in falsely confessing. The fact that they have signed releases would make it possible to prosecute them for obstructing the course of justice should this be necessary to discourage recurrence of such behaviour.

5. *Establishing the innocence or complicity of associates and friends of the criminal or patient:*—Implication of buddies and accomplices is refused for fear of being considered an informer. We suggested to one soldier who had bought a radio from a barracks-mate and was under charges for being the thief that if he submitted to narcoanalysis he might be able to give us the name of the actual thief and be absolved of being an informer. He eagerly assented, and preparations were made for his hospitalization for the procedure when the actual thief confessed.

P. V. feared the consequences of giving the names and description of the men who robbed a Post Exchange. Under narcoanalysis, in effect, he was relieved of his fear and gave excellent descriptions of the guilty men and their names, making it possible to identify them.

No less important was the emphatic and reiterated testimony of G. H. absolving a friend who was suspected of being his accomplice in the theft of butter and other foods from a warehouse at an Army post.

If we consider these suggestions from a legal standpoint, we at once see how difficult is the problem of drafting the text of rules of criminal procedure defining cases in which narcoanalysis should be permitted.

Who should rule on the application?

In view of the fact that narcoanalysis constitutes a very serious infringement of human rights, the Courts and not the public prosecutor (or in the Code Countries the juge d'instruction) should rule on the application of narcoanalysis.

E. *Suggested Limitations of Application*

W. F. Lorenz in 'Criminal Confessions under Narcosis' (*Wisconsin M. J.*, 31: 245–51, April 1932), has suggested that both the prosecution and the defendant be represented during the analytical session by legal counsel and that questions by both lawyers, or by the authorities, should be permitted, with the physician acting in an auxiliary capacity only.

It may be suggested that the prosecutor and the defendant be represented by medical experts who understand the technique of narcoanalysis and to whom an opportunity must be given to study the case history and to suggest questions. The suggestion that the physician should act in an auxiliary capacity is probably inspired by the wish to avoid conflicts of an ethical nature. Many men of the medical profession, however, are of the opinion that under these circumstances the results will be far inferior to those obtained if the physician does not act only as the instrument of opposing lawyers.

Carl P. Adatto in his above-cited article says: 'Too much questioning on the part of the examiner usually yields poor results.' He also states that the patient is again interviewed after he wakes. 'Usually he recollects little of what he said under narcosis and at times he is curious as to what occurred.'

C. T. McCormick, M.D. in the *Journal of Clin. Psychopathology*, No. 8, 1946, said, 'If adequate safeguards could be provided, the questioning of suspects under narcosis might offer possibilities for protecting the innocent and discovering the guilty.'

F. *Evaluation of Evidence*

Evidence by narcoanalysis should be corroborated by evidence from other sources.

The following case in which a French court handed down a decision as to whether the injection of pentothal should be considered as criminal assault and battery is of considerable interest. The Court of First Instance held that it was to be so considered—The Tribunal Correctionel de la Sein (Judge Durkheim) 17 Chambre, 23 Feb. 1949 (*Jrnl. Trib.* 1949, p. 301). W. Kleinermann (*Rev. intern. Dr. Pen.*, Paris 1949, p. 255) however reversed this decision.

It has been claimed that the truth drug was the instrument used in the Mindszenty and similar cases to obtain confessions. This however is not accurate. Such confessions were secured in a general environment of terror, a feeling of hopelessness being artificially created.

In actual fact, far more brutal means were used to secure the desired statements. The prisoner found himself in a position in which he would say anything required of him in order to obtain relief.

Narcoanalysis, from the time the first experiments were made in the therapeutic field, has been a controversial issue both with the legal and the medical profession. At present indications appear to point very much in the direction of the advisability of its very limited use, but it is likely that this will prove a fruitful topic for discussion for several years to come.

A SELECTIVE BIBLIOGRAPHY ON NARCOANALYSIS

ABRAHAMSON, DAVID, *Crime and the Human Mind*. New York. Columbia University Press, 1944.

Annales de Médecine Légale France, No. 44, 1945, p. 44.

Annales de Médecine Légale France, No. 4, April-May 1946.

Annales Médicopsychologiques, Tome II, No. 4. Nov. 1948. Paris. Libr. Masson et Cie.

ALTAVILLA, *Psicologia Guidiziaria*, 3rd ed. 1948.

ADAMS, E. G., 'Narcoanalysis in Private Practice' in *Dis. Nerv. System.* 6: 343–347, November 1945.

ADATTO, C. P., 'Narcoanalysis as Diagnostic aid in Criminal Cases', *Journal of Clinical Psychopathology and Psychotherapy* (Monticello, N.Y.) v. 8, Apr. 1947; pp. 721–725.

BARBARA, DOMINICK A., 'An Evaluation of the Therapeutic Role of Narcoanalysis in Mental Disorders', *Jrl. Nerv. & Ment. Dis.* 104: pp. 414–424. Oct. 1946.

BROWN, M. RALPH, *Legal Psychology: Psychology Applied to the Trial of Cases, to Crime and its Treatment, and to Mental States and Processes*. Indianapolis. The Bobbs-Merrill Co. 1926. 346 pp.

BURTT, HAROLD ERNEST, *Legal Psychology*. New York. Prentice-Hall, Inc. 1931.
Boletin de Identification y Policia Tecnica, 1947. Lima, Peru.
BOUVET, M. et GRAVEJAL, F., 'Narco-investigation et expertise psychiatrique' (*Rev. Sc. Crim. Dr. Pen. Comp.* Paris, 1948, p. 131).
BRODER, S. B., 'Sleep Induced by Sodium Amytal', *Am. Jrl. of Psychiatry*, 1936.
BARBER, T. M., 'Narco-synthesis under Sodium Amytal: Adjunct to Psychiatric diagnosis and Treatment' in *Northwest Medical Jrl.* 45: 27–30. Jan. 1946.
BLECKWENN, W. J., 'Narcosis as Therapy in Neuropsychiatric Conditions'. *Jrl. Am. Med. Assoc.* 95: 1168, 1930.
BOTSON, Interview (*Pourquoi Pas*—Janvier 1949).
BASTOS, F. DE OLIVERIRA and ARRUDA, J., 'Narcoanalysis with report of cases' in *Arq. Neuro Psiguicat*. Sao Paulo, 2: 465–470. Dec. 1944.
BULYONG, Dr. Picharn, 'Narcoanalysis': paper presented at Third International Conference, International Bar Association, Summer 1950.
CARRETERO M. FUNETE, 'Science in Identification of the Criminal' in *Vida Nueva*, 49: 3–7. January 1942.
COLLIGNON, 'Les Découvertes Dangereuses' (*Rev. Dr. Pen.* 1948/1949, p. 563).
COULHAC-MAZERIEUX (*Gaz. Pal.* Paris 21/23, Juli 1948).
DELAY, Professor JEAN, in *Le Figaro* (12 Nov. 1948, 11 Feb. 1949).
DELAY, Prof. JEAN, DESCLAUX, P. and ALJANIL, S. SHENTOUB, 'Psychosomatic Pentothal Sodium Narcoanalysis' in *Bull. Mem. Soc. Méd. de l'Hospital de Paris*. 62: 191–193, 1946.
DUPREEL, E., 'Sur l'Emploi de la Narcoanalyse comme Moyen d'Information' (*Rev. Dr. Pen*, 1948/1949, p. 566).
DUVAL, A. M., 'Narcosynthesis and Hypnotism' in *Virginia Med. Monthly* 72: 101–107, March 1945.
ELLERY, R. S., 'Psychiatry in General Practice—Treatment by Prolonged Narcosis' in *Med. Jrl. of Australia*, Nov. 23, 1940.
EY, HENRI (BONNEVAL), in *Presse Medicale*, Paris. No. 1. Janvier 1949.
FREED, H., 'Narcosynthesis of the Civilian Neurosis' *Psychiat. Quart.* 20: 39–55, January 1946.
GAGNIEUR, J. P., 'The Judicial Use of Psycho-narcosis in France', *Jrl. Crim. Law and Criminol.*, 1949. 39, 663–666.
GARRAUD, *Just. Crim.* I (207) Roux II. 73.
GERSON, MARTIN J., M.D. and VICTOROFF, VICTOR M., M.D., 'Experimental Investigation into the Validity of Confessions obtained under Sodium Amytal Narcosis', *Journal of Clinical Psychopathology*, Vol. 9, No. 3. July 1948.
GOENEN, *Strafrecht und Psychanalyse*, Breslau, 1929.
GORPHE, Tr. *l'Appréciation des Preuves en Justice*, 1947.
GRACE, HARRY A., Ass. Prof. of Psych. Univ. Ill., Urbana, Ill., UNESCO Vol. I, No. 1. Paris 1949. *Intern. Social Science Bulletin*,
GRAVEN, J., 'Le Dépistage Scientifique du Mensonge ou la Question Moderne' (*Rev. Crim. Pol. Tech.* Geneva 1948, p. 163).
GRINKER, ROY R. and SPIEGEL, JOHN P., *War Neuroses in North Africa*. New York, Josiah Macy, Jr. Foundation, 1943.

GRINKER, ROY R. and SPIEGEL, JOHN P., *War Neuroses*. Philadelphia, Blakiston Co. 1945.

HEINRICH, A., 'Attempts at Obtaining Confessions under the Effects of Anesthesia: Experiments with Ether and Evipal Sodium' in *Schmerz Narkose-Anaesth.* 11: 78–82. August 1938.

HEGER, M., 'Les Droits du Médecin Légiste' (*Rev. Dr. Pen.* 1946/1947, p. 63).

HEUVER, 'Narcoanalyse et narco-diagnostic' (*Annales Médico-Psychologiques*-Masson à Paris, April 1949.

HART, W. L., EBAUGH, F. C., and MORGAN, D. W., 'Amytal Interview', *Am. Jrl. Med. Sc.* 210. 125–131, July 1945.

HORSLEY, STEFEN, *Narcoanalysis*, London, 1943.

HOUSE, R. E., 'Scopolamine-Apomorphia Amnesia in Criminology' in *Current Research in Anesthesia.* 4: 162–9, 1925.

HOUSE, R. E., 'The Use of Scopolamine in Criminology', *Am. J. Pol. Sc.* 2: 328–336, July-August 1931.

HUYBRECHTS, G., Sérum de Vérité et Instruction Judiciaire (*Rev. Dr. Pen.* 1948–49, p. 552).

Journal of Clinical Psychopathology, Vol. 9. No. 2.

Journal of Criminal Law and Criminology, Chicago, July-August 1948. Vol. XXXIX, No. 2 and Vol. XXXVI, Sept.–Oct. 1948.

KALINOWSKY, L. B. and HOCH, H., *Shock Treatments and other Somatic Procedures in Psychiatry*. Grune and Stratton, 1946.

KAMENEVA, E. N. and YAGODKA, P. K., 'Sodium Amytal—Therapeutic and Diagnostic Uses' in the *Am. Review of Soviet Medicine* 3: 328–331. Apr. 1946.

KERR, DOUGLAS JAMES ACWORTH, *Forensic Medicine*, 4th Ed. London, A. & C. Black, 1946, 359 pp.

KLEINERMANN, W. (*Rev. Intern. Dr. Pen.* Paris 1949, p. 255).

KUBIE, L. S., 'The Use of Hypnagogic Reveries in the Recovery of Repressed Amnestic Data'. *Bull. Menninger Clin.* 7: 172–82. Sept.–Nov. 1943.

LACOMTE DU NOUY, P., *l'Homme et sa Destinée* (Paris, La Colombe, 1948, p. 93 en volg.).

La Narco-analyse à l'Académie de Médecine de Paris (Séance du 22 Mars 1949).

LEBENSOHN, Z. M., 'Shock Treatments and Narcotherapy (with Sodium Amytal)' in *Hospital Corps. Quarterly* No. 9, 18: 39–41.

Le Monde, No. 905, Paris Jeudi 25, Décembre 1947.

LENNOX, W. G., 'Real and Feigned Amnesia' (Scientific Proof and Relations of Law and Medicine) in the *Am. Jrl. of Psychiatry.* 99: 732–745. March 1943.

LEY, A., 'La Narconalyse' (*Rev. Dr. Pen.* 1948/1949, p. 548).

LEY, J., 'La Notion de Responsabilité et l'Expertise Psychiatrique' (*Rev. Dr. Pen.* 1946/1947, p. 720).

LONDON, L. S., 'Hypnosis, Hypnoanalysis and Narcoanalysis', *Am. Jrl. of Psychotherapy*. 1: 443–447, Oct. 1947.

LORENZ, W. F., 'Criminal Confessions under Narcosis', *Wisconsin M. J.* 31: 245–51, Apr. 1932.

LORENZ, W. F., 'Some Observations in Catatonia', *Psych. Quart.* 4: 95. 1930.

Luc, J., Existe-t-il un sérum de vérité? (*Science et Vie*, 1949. No. 379, p. 259).
Ludwig, Alfred O., 'Clinical Features and Diagnosis of Malingering in Military Personnel'. Use of Barbiturates as an Aid in Detection. *War. Med.* 5: 378–82 June 1944.
McCormick, C. T., 'Some Problems and Developments in the Admissibility of Confessions, *Journal of Clin. Psychopath.*, 8: 1946.
Mallinson, W. P., 'Narcoanalysis in Neuropsychiatry', *Jrl. of Royal Naval Med.* Ser. 26: 281–284. July 1940.
Manzini, *Proc. Penale* (297).
Mamel, Bernard M., *Jrl. of Criminal Law and Criminology*, XXXVI. No. 2. Jul/Aug. 1945.
Marshall, S. V., 'Pentothal Sodium; Use under War Conditions', *Med. Jrl. of Australia*, 2: 694–700. March 1942.
Mezger, Ed., *Die Bedeutung der Psychanalyse fuer die Rechtspflege*, 1933.
Millan, Alfonso, 'El Narcoanalisis en el Derecho Procesal Penal.' (Narcoanalysis in Lawful Penal Process). *Criminalia. Mex.* 1948, 14, pp. 440–456.
Monde du Travail, Lundi, 27 January 1947.
Muehlberger, C. W., 'Criminal Confessions under Narcosis', *J. Crim. Law & Criminology* 26: 449–51, 1935.
Mullins, Claud., *Crime and Psychology*. London, Methuen, 1943, 234 pp.
Muris, D. P., 'Intravenous Barbiturates as an Aid in Diagnosis and Treatment of Conversion Hysteria and Malingering'. *Mil. Surgeon* 96; 509–13, July 1945.
—— and Margolin, S., 'The Therapeutic Value of Drugs in the Process of Repression Dissociation and Synthesis'. *Psychosom. Med.* 7: 147–51, May 1945.
Poignard, 'Narcoanalyse et sérum de vérité' (*Hommes et Mondes*, Octobre 1948).
Reik, Theodor, *The Unknown Murderer*. New York, Prentice Hall, 1945.
Revue de Criminologie et de Police Technique, Genève, July–Sept. 1948, Vol. II.
Revue Internationale de Criminalistique, Lyon 1934, No. 3.
Revue de Droit Pénal et de Criminologie, Brussels, Belgium, Nov. 1947.
Revue International de Police Criminelle, 4 Année. No. 29, June–July 1949.
Reznikoff, L., 'Narcoanalysis and Narco-Synthesis (with Sodium Amytal or Pentothal)' in *Hebrew Medical Jrl.* 1: 182, 1947.
Robin, J., 'Pentothal, Drogue de l'Aveu' (*Etudes*) Oct. 1948.
Robinson, H. M., *La Science contre le Crime*, Paris, Payot, 1941.
Rousselet, M., 'Les Ruses et les Artifices dans l'Instruction Criminelle' (*Rev. Sc. Crim. Dr. Pen. Comp.* Paris 1946, p. 50).
Saher, Dr. Edward V., *Narcoanalysis*, Paper presented at Third International Conference, International Bar Association, London, July, 1950.
Sargent, W., and Slater, E., 'Acute War Neuroses'. *Lancet* 2: 1, 1940.

SASSERATH, S., 'La Justice Françoise et l'emploi du Pentothal' (*Rev. Intern. Pol. Crim.* 1949, No. 29 and *Rev. Dr. Pen.* 1948/1949, p. 962).

SASSERATH, S., *Rev. Dr. Pen.* 1948/1949, p. 871 and *Jrl. Trib.* 1949, p. 410.

SCHNEIDER, PIERRE B. (U. Basel Switzerland) 'Psychiatrie Légale et Narcoanalyse' (Legal Psychiatry and Narcoanalysis), *Schweiz. Arch. Neurol. Psychiat.* 1948, 62, 352–371.

SCHOENKE, Prof. Dr. A., *Grenzen des Sachverstaendigen Beweises*, D. R. 2, 49: 203.

SMITH, H. W., 'Scientific Proof and Relations of Law and Medicine' in *Annals of International Medicine.* 18: 450–490. April 1943. Also in *Clinics* 1: 1353–1404, April 1943.

SMITH, SYDNEY, *Forensic Medicine*. Boston, Little Brown & Co. 1949.

SPACCARELLI, G. and CERQUETELLI, G., 'Narcoanalysis and Narco-suggestion' in *Clin. Nuova.* 2: 188–196. April 1946.

STEENWINKEL, F. L. M., 'Chemodiagnosis in Psychiatry by means of Barbiturate Narcosis' in the *Nederl. Tijdschr. v. Geneesk.* 90: 1514–1518. Oct. 26, 1946.

SULLIVAN, D. J., 'Psychiatric Uses of Intravaneous Sodium Amytal' in. *Am. Jrl. of Psychiatry.* 99: 411–418. Nov. 1942.

STRYKER, LLOYD PAUL, *Courts and Doctors*, New York. The MacMillan Company, 1932.

SWARTHOUT, J. A., 'Sodium Pentothal: Properties and Uses'. *Jrl. of Am. Inst. of Homeopathology.* 39: 227–230. July 1946.

TAHON, R., 'La liberté Individuelle et un Nouveau Procédé d'Expertise Mentale' (*Rev. Dr. Pen.* 1947/1948; pp. 113–140).

Thesis International Centrum voor Sociaal Verweer (*Riv. di Difesa Sociale*, Genova, (Italy) 1947/1948/1949).

TRAIN, Dr. GEORGE J., *Handbook of Correctional Psychology* 1947.

—— 'Truth Serum or Scopolamine in Interrogation of Criminal Suspects'. *Hygeia* 10: 337–40, April 1932.

VABRES, H. DONNEDIEU DE, *La Justice Françoise et l'Emploi du Pentothal*, Paris, 1949.

VABRES, H. DONNEDIEU de, *Traité de droit Criminol. Procédure Crim.* (Paris, Sirey, 1947), pp. 7188–7189.

VERSELE, S. C., 'Het Wetenschappelijk Trachten naar Bewijs', in *Rechtskundig Weekblad*, Sept. 18/49 13e Jaargang No. 1.

WILBUR, C. B., 'Uses of Barbiturates Intravenously in Neuropsychiatry' in *Disorders of the Nervous System.* 5: 293. Oct. 369. Dec. 1944.

WILDE, J. F., 'Narcoanalysis in the Treatment of war neuroses'. *Brit. Med. J.* 2: 4, 1942.

YOTIS, Dr. CHRISTO P., *Narcoanalysis*, Athens, 1949.

YOTIS, Dr. CHRISTO P., 'La Narcoanalyse en Justice Pénale', Paper presented to Third International Conference, International Bar Association, London, July, 1950.

MAR 18 1998

FEB 16 1999
JUN 1 1 2002